13306

KT-475-834

ɔital,

**a**ccess to
**C**linical
**e**ducation

# Pressure Sores

*For Churchill Livingstone:*

*Commissioning Editor:* Ellen Green
*Project Manager:* Valerie Burgess
*Project Development Editor:* Mairi McCubbin
*Designer:* Judith Wright
*Illustrator:* Robert Britton
*Copy-editor:* Sue Beasley
*Page Layout:* Kate Walshaw
*Indexer:* Liza Weinkove
*Sales Promotion Executive:* Hilary Brown

# access to
# Clinical
# education

# Pressure
# Sores

## Jenny Phillips

BSc(Hons) DipN RGN

Nurse Tutor, Faculty of Nursing and Health Studies,
Taranaki Polytechnic, New Plymouth, New Zealand
Formerly Tissue Viability Adviser,
Lincolnshire District Healthcare Trust, Lincoln, UK


*Educational Consultant, Access to Clinical Education series*
## Diane Marks-Maran

BSc RGN DipN(Lond) RNT

Associate Director, Wolfson Institute for Health Sciences, and
Head of the Centre for Teaching and Learning in Health Sciences,
Thames Valley University, London, UK

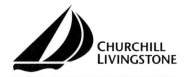

CHURCHILL
LIVINGSTONE

NEW YORK EDINBURGH LONDON MELBOURNE SAN FRANCISCO AND TOKYO 1997

CHURCHILL LIVINGSTONE

Medical Division of Pearson Professional Limited
Distributed in the United States of America by Churchill Livingstone Inc.,
650 Avenue of the Americas, New York, N.Y. 10011, and by associated
companies, branches and representatives throughout the world.

First edition 1997

ISBN 0 443 05532 7

**British Library of Cataloguing in Publication Data**
A catalogue record for this book is available from the British Library.

**Library of Congress Cataloging in Publication Data**
A catalogue record for this book is available from the Library of Congress

Medical knowledge is constantly changing. As new information becomes
available, changes in treatment, procedures, equipment and the use of
drugs become necessary. The editors/authors/contributors and the
publishers have, as far as it is possible, taken care to ensure that the
information given in this text is accurate and up to date. However,
readers are strongly advised to confirm that the information, especially
with regard to drug usage, complies with latest legislation and and
standards of practice.

The
publisher's
policy is to use
**paper manufactured
from sustainable forests**

Produced by Longman Singapore Publishers Pte Ltd
Printed in Singapore

# Contents

# Preface

Despite many advances in the world of medicine, pressure sores remain a major problem, causing suffering to patients and increasing health care costs. There are still uncertainties about the importance of different contributory factors, the type and duration of pressures applied, and their effects on development and prevention of pressure sores.

It is widely accepted that a multi-disciplinary team approach is the way forward, and this book advocates such an approach for policy formation and wound formularies. However, the reality is that nurses are at the forefront of prevention and treatment of pressure sores in the majority of health care settings. This book was written to help nurses in any care setting with some of the many problems relating to prevention and treatment of pressure sores.

Many nurses do not have easy access to study days and specialised courses, for a variety of reasons. This book is one of a new series of open learning texts, called 'Access to Clinical Education' (ACE), enabling nursing staff to study in their own time and at their chosen level. (For more information about the series see 'About the series' on page 1.)

The aim of this book is to:

- provide a comprehensive knowledge of the effects of pressure and shear forces on the tissues
- highlight sources of expertise available to help nursing staff
- encourage nurses to look at ways of auditing and changing their own practice, and introducing research-based care

- provide an overview of some of the potential problems relating to the move to primary health care.

The areas that cause most confusion and debate among clinical staff are covered in specific sections, as follows:

- pressure-relieving equipment
- risk assessment scores
- grading of pressure sores
- wound care in relation to pressure sores.
  (For more comprehensive study of wound care, see *Wound Management* in this series.)

This book is based on wide experience as a nurse specialist, working directly with clinical staff in acute care settings, the community and the private sectors, and in identifying the constantly recurring problems encountered in all areas. I hope that the clinical focus adopted in the books in the Access to Clinical Education series (ACE), will encourage more staff to study, to achieve their own goals and then to look at ways of improving care for patients in their own care settings.

New Zealand, 1997                                                    J.L.P.

NB Some of the activities may require verbal or written consent from patients, to comply with privacy laws relating to the individual person.

# Acknowledgements

The author would like to thank her husband for his patience and support during the writing of this and while undertaking further studies.

The publishers would like to thank Kate Davies, University Hospital of Wales, Cardiff and Jenny Jepson, Thames Valley University, London, for acting as Critical Readers for this book; and the Community and District Nursing Association for their assistance in field testing the books in the ACE series.

We are also grateful to the following for permission to reproduce the following articles in the Reader:

Journal of Tissue Viability for Reader 3—Oliver E 1994 Maintaining nutritional support in the community. Journal of Tissue Viability 4(1): 28–32

Lippincott-Raven for Reader 15—Breu C, Dracup K 1976 Implementing nursing research in a critical care setting. Journal of Nursing Administration December 1976: 14–17

Macmillan Magazines Ltd for: Reader 1—O'Dea 1993 Prevalence of pressure damage in hospital patients in the UK. Journal of Wound Care 2(4): 223–225; Reader 2—Pinchofsky-Devin G 1994 Nutrition and wound healing. Journal of Wound Care 3(5): 232–233; Reader 4—Pressure-relieving/reducing mattresses. Journal of Wound Care 1995 4(9): 410–411; Reader 6 —Evans V, Fear M 1992 John's story. Community Outlook March 1992; Reader 7—Charalambous L 1995 Development of the link-nurse role in clinical settings. Nursing Times 91(11): 36–37; Reader 9— Baroness Masham of Ilton 1994 Healing: a patient's perspective. Journal of Wound Care 3(4): 195–196; Reader 10—Rough M, Brooks H The prevention of pressure sores after hospital discharge. Community Nurse May 1995: 27–28; Reader 11—Vernon D 1991 Pressure sore success. Journal of Wound Care/ Nursing Times 87(49); Reader 12—Rithalia S V S, Moore E 1994 The use of an airwave mattress for pressure relief. Journal of Wound Care 3(4): 171–173; Reader 13—Phillips S, Frost J 1993 A barrier to continuity of care. Professional Nurse Wound Care on FP10 May 1993: 536–542 Reader 14—Elliott M 1995 Care management in the community: a case study. Nursing Times 91(48): 34–35; Reader 16—Devon S The nurse formulary and benefits in practice. Nurse Prescriber, Community Nurse: 8–10; Reader 17— Field G 1993 Practice themes. Nursing Times 89(49)

North Lincolnshire Health Authority for Reader 5 —Preston K W Positioning for Comfort and Pressure Relief.

# About the series  *Diane Marks-Maran*

This book has been designed to enable nurses to improve their specialist knowledge and understanding of an important area of clinical practice. To help you to make the most of this learning package, we have designed this introductory section as a guideline for those of you who are new to open and distance learning.

## Who is this book for?

This book is for nurses in either hospital or community settings, or in the private sector, who provide wound care to a variety of patients or clients and who want to take the opportunity, through this learning package, to ensure that their knowledge and skills are up to date and that their practice is evidence based.

## What is the best way for me to use this learning package?

This depends upon what you want to gain from completing the package. At one level, this book is an excellent way to update your clinical knowledge and skill through open learning. Open learning means that you complete the package in your own time and at your own pace, taking as long as you like, reading selectively from the text and focusing on those aspects that are important to you. You complete no assessment and merely complete the activities within the package for your own interest.

At another level, in addition to updating clinical knowledge and skill, you may wish to complete this book as part of fulfilling your PREP requirements. In this case, you will need to show evidence in your professional portfolio of how this package has improved your clinical practice.

At a third level, as well as updating your clinical knowledge and skill, you may be planning to undertake further study at your local university to gain, for example, a post-registration qualification and a further academic award. In this case, completing this package and successfully passing the written assessment at the end of the book may be used to gain academic credits towards your planned academic award if the university of your choice has approved this programme of study.

## What do the learning outcomes mean?

More and more, colleges and universities are aware of the need to make explicit the exact requirements for completing a module or programme successfully. Learning outcomes are one way of doing this.

Learning outcomes indicate the specific knowledge, skills and understandings you will be exposed to in the learning package. They also tell you what your assessment will entail. Additionally, if you are planning to use this book towards achieving your PREP professional requirements, you may find the learning outcomes a useful basis for submitting evidence of learning within your personal professional profile.

## What do I need to do to complete this book for my PREP requirements?

Completing this book can be used towards fulfilment of your PREP requirements to show evidence of your continued learning. The UKCC has sent you a package of information entitled 'PREP and You' which explains how to complete a personal professional profile to show evidence of learning and improvement in practice. If you have not received this information, the UKCC will be happy to send you the package. In addition, issue 17 of the UKCC magazine *Register* (Summer 1996) gives a comprehensive guide to writing your personal professional profile. Completing the written assessment at the end of this book provides one piece of evidence you can include in your profile even if you do not submit it for marking to gain academic credits; recording your reflection on learning as a result of completing this package is another form of evidence to include in your profile.

## What do I need to do if I want to gain academic credits for completing this book?

Some universities have accredited this learning package at both diploma level (level 2) and degree level (level 3). Accreditation has been awarded on the basis of the expected learning outcomes for the package and for the written assessment at the end of the package. You can only receive academic credits for completing the written assessment and achieving a pass grade for that assessment. You can receive academic credits at level 2 if you successfully pass the associated assessment and achieve the level 2 learning outcomes; you will receive level 3 credits if you successfully pass the level 3 assessment at the end of the package and achieve the associated learning outcomes. This means that you can use this package towards your future study to gain a Diploma in Higher Education in Nursing or a BSc in nursing.

Prior to undertaking the assessment, you should find out from the university of your choice whether they will accredit this learning pack. If they have done so, you will be able, for a registration fee, to submit your assessment for marking. If you successfully pass the assessment, you will get the credits that your university has chosen to award this learning package. Thames Valley University (TVU) has already accredited this package and would be willing to undertake this service for you. Other universities will follow shortly. The university of your choice may, however, accept the credits awarded you by institutions such as TVU through their APL/APEL process. A visual illustration of how to use this learning package is given in Figure 1.

## What exactly does level 2 study mean?

When we talk about a package or course being at level 2 or level 3 it means that the work expected of you is assessed at a certain level. Level 2 normally equates to the second year of a full-time degree programme, at the end of which students would achieve a Diploma in Higher Education. However, modern education allows students to take various routes, including part-time and distance learning modes.

At level 2 you are expected to:

- demonstrate good understanding of relevant concepts and issues
- make appropriate use and application of relevant research
- demonstrate the ability to solve problems
- analyse a range of information and apply this knowledge to practice
- demonstrate the ability to construct arguments and evaluate the relevance of issues to your professional practice.

Level 2 means that you are expected to demonstrate the ability to collect information and apply that information to solve a simple but unpredictable problem or a complex but predictable problem in your practice. Level 2 also means that you are

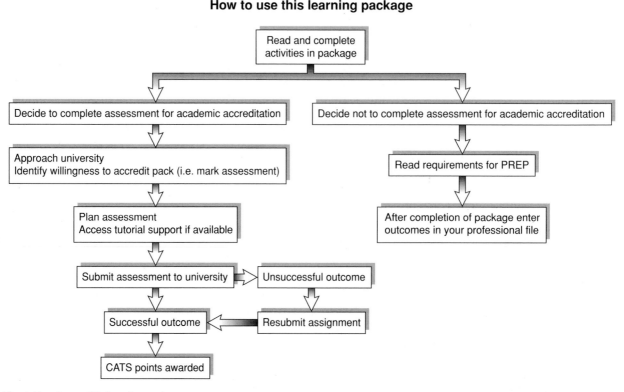

**How to use this learning package**

**Fig. 1** How to use this learning package.

expected to manage care within broad guidelines for defined activities and to demonstrate knowledge and understanding of the subject and the variety of ideas and frameworks which may be applied to this subject. A level 2 student is one who also demonstrates the ability to analyse a variety of types of information with minimum guidance, can apply major theories of discipline and can compare alternative methods or techniques for gathering data. Within a level 2 learning package you will show that you can use a range of ideas and information towards a given purpose, such as solving a particular patient problem or situation, and can select appropriate techniques of evaluation, demonstrating that you are able to evaluate the relevance and significance of information you have collected.

In addition, when given a complex task to undertake, a level 2 student should demonstrate that she or he can choose an appropriate set of actions in sequence to complete the task, and can evaluate individual performance in terms of strengths and weaknesses. Level 2 students can challenge received opinion, adopt flexible approaches to study, identify their own learning needs and undertake activities to improve their own performance. At level 2 you are expected to demonstrate that you can study autonomously in completing straightforward study tasks. In tackling problems you should demonstrate that you can identify the key elements of a problem and choose appropriate methods for resolving problems.

## What does level 3 study mean?

Level 3 study refers to a range of more advanced academic skills and equates to the third year of a full-time degree course. In addition to level 2 skills you are expected to:

- demonstrate a comprehensive and detailed knowledge of a major subject area
- critically analyse new or abstract information and relate this to your professional practice
- design creative solutions to problems
- critically evaluate evidence which supports conclusions or recommendations
- demonstrate the ability to sustain analytical argument whilst being aware of controversies and critical standpoints
- demonstrate the ability to develop a constructive, independent and original line of thought.

At level 3, you are expected to be able to demonstrate that you can work with complex and unpredictable situations, apply a wide range of innovative and standard techniques and demonstrate autonomy in planning and managing resources within broad guidelines. Your written assessments at level 3 should show that you can incorporate awareness of personal

responsibility and a critical ethical dimension into your written work. A level 3 student demonstrates a comprehensive and detailed knowledge of a major subject area with the ability to demonstrate specialisation and yet realise that knowledge within a specialism is always growing and changing. A level 3 student can analyse new and/or abstract data without guidance and can transform abstracted data and concepts towards a given purpose with minimum guidance. In addition, a level 3 student can also design novel solutions to problems and can critically evaluate evidence which supports conclusions or recommendations. The students can select appropriate responses to a situation from a repertoire of actions and can evaluate their own performance and the performance of others.

In addition, people who are working at level 3 can manage their own learning using a wide range of resources, can seek and make use of feedback and can apply their own criteria for judging their performance. Problem solving at level 3 involves demonstrating confidence and flexibility in identifying and defining complex problems and applying appropriate knowledge and evidence to their solutions.

## I have never studied using an independent method before. How can I get help in developing the study skills I need to work in this way?

Studying independently through open and distance learning is very different from taking a course at a college or university. It affords nurses the opportunity to study at their own pace, in their own environment and in their own time. Distance learning is especially beneficial for nurses who do not have access to a university-based course, owing to geographical, work or domestic constraints or situations. However, studying through open or distance learning does require good study skills and time-management skills to make the most of the learning package. We would recommend that you read one of the many guides to study skills which are available for students. This will give you practical advice on how to get the most out of learning packages such as this one. We particularly recommend the following two books:

- Goodall C 1995 *A Survivor's Guide to Study Skills and Student Assessments*. Churchill Livingstone, Edinburgh
- Parnell J, Kendrick K 1994 *Study Skills for Nurses*. Churchill Livingstone, Edinburgh.

In addition, study skills packs may be available from the university accrediting the package; tutorial support may also be offered. Thames Valley University is able to provide learning support in the form of feedback, tutorial support and advice to nurses undertaking this book. Details of the type of learning and tutorial support available from TVU, as well as the amount and cost, are available from:

Jean Clayton
APL Manager
Wolfson School of Health Sciences
Thames Valley University
32–38 Uxbridge Road
London W5 2BS
Tel: 0181 280 5230
Fax: 0181 280 5125
e-mail: jean.clayton@tvu.ac.uk

## What types of learning activities will I be undertaking in this book?

In order to make this book interesting and varied, the authors have included a wide range of activities for you to complete. One type is reading activities. These are interesting and informative parts of the package which are designed to give you important information and knowledge about the subject. Sometimes a reading activity will request that you read an article from a journal on a particular subject or aspect of care. This article can be found in the Reader at the back of the book. Reading activities are often followed by self-assessment questions (SAQs). SAQs are designed to enable you to test your understanding of what you have read and draw together some of the important points in the reading you have just completed. Sometimes SAQs are included to assess your prior learning (e.g. one SAQ might ask you to write your own definition of a wound) or are in the form of short true/false questions.

Another type of activity in the package is that which asks you to describe something that currently happens in your own practice. You may be asked to reflect on some previous experience or patient. This may be followed by a feedback section where the author enables you to analyse your practice or previous experience against the literature, research and evidence. Another activity may ask you to look at a photograph and make certain observations. This will be followed by some kind of feedback to check your observations with those of the author. Other activities may include completing a chart or diagram, followed by feedback from the author of the package.

As you can see, undertaking a learning package is not the same thing as reading a book! It involves you in a wide variety of activities to find information, use information, analyse information and make clinical judgements. You will always be given some sort of feedback from the activities within the package.

## You mentioned a Reader at the end of this package. What is it?

The Reader is a selection of articles from various professional journals about the subject you are studying in the learning package. We recognise that some nurses are undertaking distance learning study because they do not have easy access to a college or university in their geographical area and therefore may not have access to some of the journals which specialise in the subject of this learning package. For this reason, we are including a Reader within the book. Some of the learning activities within the package ask you to read certain articles from the Reader and answer questions about those articles. Other articles are just related to the subject and are useful for you to have as reference material and to help you complete your written assessment.

## There seem to be a lot of terms used in this book. How can I be sure that I am understanding these terms in the way I am supposed to?

To help you understand the terminology in this book the following glossary will be helpful.

**Critically analyse.** To critically analyse something means to look at a wide range of information about a subject or issue, to identify the strengths and weaknesses of the arguments for or against something, draw conclusions based on the diverse information available to you and defend your conclusions with reference to the widest possible sources of information. At level 2, students should be able to analyse a range of information with minimum guidance, apply major theories of a discipline and compare alternative methods or techniques for obtaining data (SEEC 1996). Level 3 critical analysis means that students can analyse new and/or abstract data and situations without guidance using a wide range of techniques appropriate to the subject being studied (SEEC 1996).

**Define.** When you are asked to define something in a learning activity, what you are being asked to do is to write the meaning of something, e.g. a wound is ….

**Demonstrate knowledge.** Demonstrating knowledge involves showing that you know relevant facts, principles and concepts and that you can select these appropriately to make a clinical decision and justify that decision. Knowledge is demonstrated by defining, naming, listing or identifying parts of a whole as well as interpreting information through explaining and describing facts and applying facts to solve a problem or to give an example of a situation.

**Describe.** When you are asked to describe something, you are being asked to interpret information. This means that you must first show that you have the information and then give your interpretation of it.

**Evaluate.** Evaluating involves assessing or re-assessing a situation, criticising it, identifying strengths and weaknesses, discriminating or judging something. In nursing, evaluation often involves making a judgement of care given as compared to evidence or research.

**Reflect.** Reflection is thinking in a structured way in order to learn something from your experiences as a nurse and to make a decision or take an action as a result of your thinking. There are a number of frameworks for reflection, each of which offers structured questions to think through a situation and learn from it. At the end of structured reflection is some sort of learning which points you in new directions for the way you practise as a nurse.

## When I complete the activities in this book and write my assessment, how should I reference my essay?

It is important to cite references appropriately. There are a number of ways of referencing and, so long as you select a recognised method and are consistent in your approach, it does not matter which one you use. You should seek guidance from the university who will be marking your assessment about their preferred referencing system. Details of some approaches to referencing can be found in the two study skills books which were identified earlier.

REFERENCE

SEEC 1996 Guidelines on levels and generic levels descriptors. South East England Consortium/Wales HE CATS

# Introduction

The problem of pressure sores is timeless. Despite increasingly sophisticated technology enabling us to diagnose and treat disease, few problems develop so quickly, persist so tenaciously and heal so slowly as the pressure sore. In addition, perhaps no other problem is so directly seen as a reflection of the quality of nursing care the patient has received.

Pajk et al 1989

This quotation sums up the ongoing problem of pressure sores and the fact that they are still seen as a nursing problem despite all the knowledge which has been and is being discovered relating to:

- how they start
- who is susceptible to them
- how to prevent them
- how to treat them once they have occurred.

All nurses have some knowledge of pressure sores, but can you answer the following questions?

- Which forces contribute to pressure sores, and what is the effect that they have on the skin and microcirculation?
- How do different types of pressure relieving equipment work?
- How do different types of dressings work?
- What is your legal position if a patient in your care develops pressure damage?

This book aims to answer these and many more questions, in the hope that improved quality of patient care and changes in practice may result from the nurses who have completed this unit of study.

# Learning outcomes

## LEVEL 2 LEARNING OUTCOMES

At the end of this book nurses will demonstrate that they can:

1. explain and discuss in depth the scope and nature of the problem of pressure sores, their causes, risk factors and how they can be prevented
2. critically analyse the assessment, treatment and support given to patients who are either at risk from pressure sores or who have an established pressure sore.

## LEVEL 3 LEARNING OUTCOMES

At the end of this book nurses will demonstrate that they can:

1. critically evaluate one aspect of pressure sore prevention, management or support provided in your practice area and the extent to which practice reflects the literature
2. plan a change in your own practice setting related to pressure sore prevention or management taking into account research evidence, government targets, local and/or national guidelines and/or technological advances.

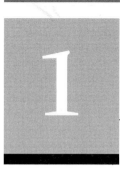

# Influencing factors

## LEARNING OUTCOMES

At the end of this section you will be able to:

- give an overview of how prevention and treatment of pressure sores have progressed since they were first recognised
- discuss the impact that demographic changes are likely to have on the prevalence of pressure sores
- identify the different societies with a role in working towards improving the situation.

A pressure sore has been described by Collier (1995) as 'ulceration of the skin due to damage caused by prolonged pressure', although he also acknowledges that other causes exist. Clarke (1988) says that pressure upon the soft tissues is the most important cause, while Rough (1994) identifies a combination of factors, including pressure, shear and friction. At its most severe, a pressure sore is an area of tissue which has died from a lack of oxygen resulting from pressure and disruption to the blood supply, but also termed as pressure sores are areas showing early signs of tissue damage, where intervention can often prevent full tissue death occurring. This is discussed in more detail in Section 2.

## 1.1 HISTORICAL PERSPECTIVE

It is a sad but true fact that much nursing and medical care is based on myth and ritual (Walsh & Ford 1989), and nowhere is this more apparent than in pressure sore prevention and management. It is probably true to say that, because of increasing awareness of the problem, the last 20 years has seen more progress than had occurred previously. A quick look at the history of pressure sore prevention and wound management will help to explain some of the rituals, but not why they have persisted for so long.

### Pressure sore prevention

There have been reports of pressure sores on mummies (Thompson Rowling 1961), and they were first intimated in the literature in the 16th century, with further accounts in the 17th century, so they are certainly not a new phenomenon. The first person to try to analyse the cause of pressure sores was Charcot (1877). He looked at patients suffering from nerve damage and spinal cord injuries, recognising that they were the most often afflicted. He recognised immobility and anaesthesia of the affected area as prime factors, but put pressure as a secondary cause. He also identified the following characteristics:

- pressure sores were usually found on the sacrum
- they often became infected and were dangerous to the patient
- skin changes occurred which pointed to a pressure sore developing
- maceration from urine seepage increased the problem
- they could appear within 2 days, hence his name for them of ominous sores.

It seems amazing therefore to realise that not until the 1940s was it recognised that bladder care and turning patients contributed to reducing the number of pressure sores which developed, because much of Charcot's work was previously ignored.

Nurses were at the forefront of pressure sore prevention, and indeed pressure sores were often assumed to be a result of defective nursing care (Versluysen 1985). In the late 1960s and early 1970s there were still pressure sore books, in which every patient developing a sore had to be recorded and reported to Matron, which earned a black mark for those who were on the shift when the sore occurred, and many nursing staff around now can still remember these. This was before a greater understanding of the many factors involved was achieved, and indeed today there are still things not fully understood, such as why one of two seemingly identical patients will develop a pressure sore and the other will not. Nurses attempted to solve this problem, which carried with it much guilt for the staff, by trying to prevent the skin breakdown using various methods such as:

- softening the skin—oil or creams rubbed in
- hardening the skin—methylated spirits, alcohol
- rubbing the skin to get the circulation going again.

Using methylated spirits or oil actually promotes skin breakdown and destroys the normal skin flora and pH balance, providing a pathway for infection (Walsh & Ford 1989). Walsh & Ford also state that 'no agent applied to the skin has been demonstrated to reduce the incidence of pressure sores'.

Despite the findings in the 1940s that turning and bladder control had a crucial role to play, and work done in 1962 by Norton et al which showed that turning the patients and not applying alcohol to the skin reduced the percentage of patients with pressure damage from 25 to 9, Anthony (1987) recorded some of the measures listed above still being used at a time when they were known not only to be ineffective but to increase the risk of damage. This represented ritualised care in the face of research-based findings, but how many nurses know why they carry out some of the procedures that they do?

## Activity                    15 MINUTES

Look at Table 1.1 which lists some of the methods used to prevent pressure sores from developing, then in the columns tick whether you have used any of them in the last 5 years, and tick the reasons why you used them. See whether you can identify any problems with your answers and why.

## FEEDBACK

You should only have been using the second and third options when trying to relieve pressure, because research has shown the first and fourth to be inefficient and harmful.

The only reason you should be using any of the methods is because you know there is research to back up their use.

## Wound care

Evidence exists of wound care in Egypt, and indeed this was when cloth was used in the form of linen, usually combined with honey and grease. Strips of linen were placed over the wound and honey and grease spread on top (Knight 1985). This is interesting as it would have created a moist environment at the wound surface, which has proved to be the most beneficial for wound healing, yet wound healing went through many more stages before returning to this concept. Winter (1962) provided the research findings which form the basis of present-day wound management and moist wound healing, when he discovered that pigs he was experimenting on healed quicker when their wounds were covered with cling film, than those whose wounds were more conventionally covered. Wounds in the early days were mostly war wounds or accidents, and these were covered with a variety of substances such as:

- animal dung
- honey
- tar
- leaves
- oils
- cobwebs.

A major setback to wound care occurred in late Roman times, when Galen identified that many wounds had pus, and concluded that this was essential for wound healing to occur (Knight 1985). This became known as the laudable pus theory and, despite the attempts of some people to discredit it, it persisted right through until the work of Pasteur and Lister in the late 19th century. It meant that many patients, particularly those with war wounds, were subjected to horrific measures to make their wounds ooze pus if they did not already do so, an

| Table 1.1 | | | | |
| --- | --- | --- | --- | --- |
| Method | Used in last 5 years | Because you were told to | Because it had been proved effective by recent research | Because you had always done it that way |
| Rubbing the skin when you turn the patient | | | | |
| Turning the patient 2-hourly | | | | |
| Trying to relieve pressure being applied to patient | | | | |
| Applying: | | | | |
| —creams | | | | |
| —talcum powder | | | | |
| —spirits | | | | |

example being insertion of oil into the wound site. With the advent of Pasteur (antisepsis) and Lister (asepsis) came the first forerunner of modern dressings, tulle gras.

Because of the lack of interest shown by the medical establishment in the care of chronic wounds such as pressure sores and leg ulcers, wound care moved into the domain of nurses (Bennett & Moody 1995), and so nurses developed it as one of their own areas. More recently, as the medical profession has tried to reclaim this area, there have been conflicts, none greater than the Eusol debate, which has little to do with the effects of the solution and everything to do with who holds the reins of power in wound care. Outdated ritualistic practices continued to be used, for example egg white and oxygen. The only way to supply oxygen to the wound for healing is via the capillaries. In 1985 Gould found that out of 28 ward sisters treating pressure sores, only 5 were relieving the pressure, indicating a lack of understanding of what was causing the wound. The fact remains that nurses continue to deal with the majority of chronic wounds and, while there are members of both the nursing and medical professions whose knowledge base is not as good as it could be, there are experts in both fields whose knowledge should be respected across professional boundaries. Combining this knowledge into multidisciplinary teamwork provides the basis for high quality patient care.

## Self-assessment    15 MINUTES

Answer the following questions to test your understanding of what you have read so far.

1. Who first tried to analyse pressure sores in detail and in which year?
2. What key factors did he recognise in relation to them?
3. What was the first wound dressing to promote moist wound healing?
4. What are the biggest blocks to progress in both the areas discussed?

## FEEDBACK

1 & 2. You should have given the answers that Charcot was the first to analyse pressure sores in 1877 and that immobility and anaesthesia were the prime causes recognised by him. He noted that the sores were usually sacral and easily infected, skin changes indicated their formation,

urine seepage made things worse, and they could appear within 2 days.
3. You should have said that honey and grease in Egyptian times was the first dressing to promote moist wound healing.
4. The biggest block to progress is continued reliance on ritualistic practice and lack of knowledge of new research-based techniques.

## 1.2 DEMOGRAPHIC CHANGES

While attempts are being made to set reduction targets for the numbers of people developing pressure sores (see Sect. 2), it is likely that demographic changes which are occurring may have an effect on whether or not these can be achieved.

In 1983 David et al undertook a survey of 20 health districts covering four regional authorities, and found that 85% of patients with pressure sores were over 65 years of age. Age in itself does not cause pressure damage, but combined with illness it is a major problem. Bennett & Moody (1995) recognise that the elderly are more likely to have multiple illnesses and spend longer in hospitals, while Harding et al (1993) report that 70% of patients over 75 have long-standing illnesses. In a survey which looked at 3213 patients in hospital, O'Dea (1993; Reader Article 1) found that 18.6% of patients suffered from pressures sores and, of these, 44% were over the age of 70 years. One of the biggest risk groups is elderly patients with fractured femurs (Versluysen 1986). Many of the elderly also suffer from malnutrition, or at least reduced nutritional intake (Oliver 1994) which also predisposes to pressure damage. Section 3 looks in more detail at why all these increase the risk of pressure sore development. An additional fact is that the elderly heal more slowly than younger people (Harding et al 1993), so once an elderly person has a wound it is likely to be a chronic one resulting in more problems for patient and carers.

## Activity    15 MINUTES

Article 1 in the Reader (p. 106) contains some relevant observations relating to age and pressure sore development. Read the article and then answer the following questions.

1. Which group of patients is most likely to develop pressure damage?
2. Of the total number of patients with pressure damage what percentage comes into this group?

## FEEDBACK

1. You should have said that O'Dea found that the group of people most likely to develop pressure sores were those over 70 years of age.
2. Out of the 598 patients with pressure damage, 66.4% were over 70 years of age.

Population forecasts for the next 40–50 years show that the total population growth will slow down, but with improvements in lifestyle and increase in medical interventions both the over-65 and the over-85 age groups will get bigger as people live longer (Harding et al 1993). As these people require health care for medical or surgical reasons, so their risk of developing pressure sores will rise. There is also the issue of who will care for them in their old age. Another change which is occurring is the breakdown of the family unit, and many elderly people find themselves alone or with one carer who is also elderly and unable to do much in the way of turning or moving them, one of the accepted prevention strategies (Collier 1995).

The Community Care Act 1990 is likely to result in a greater number of highly dependent people being cared for in their own homes (Caldock 1993). Caldock also points out that social services take the lead role in assessment for social needs for the care of the elderly, along with a budget which covers social but not health needs. However, before this system works effectively, more needs to be done towards multidisciplinary care and provision of resources to solve the escalating problem of caring for the elderly in their own homes. As more home carers take on the burden of patients, sometimes without full support and resources, there is likely to be an increase in the number of pressure sores which develop at home, particularly if the patients there are older and more frail than previously. Another issue here is again related to the findings of O'Dea (1993) that although more pressure sores started in hospital than in other care settings, the majority of deep ones came from outside the hospital. With the increase in the elderly population, this must be an area that needs looking at urgently if major pressure sore problems are not to arise. Authorities need to know where in the community pressure sores start so that they can target these areas by education and provision of more resources if necessary.

## Activity                          1–2 HOURS

Before completing this activity, obtain permission from your manager to carry out the exercise which comprises a small patient audit. To ensure confidentiality, give each patient a number instead of using his or her name. Select three to six patients in your care with pressure sores, whether superficial or deep. Using the medical and nursing notes, and by talking to the patients, answer the questions in Table 1.2 and fill in the table. As you complete the columns, you may see some interesting patterns emerging.

| Table 1.2 | | | | | | | |
| --- | --- | --- | --- | --- | --- | --- | --- |
| Question | Patient 1 | Patient 2 | Patient 3 | Patient 4 | Patient 5 | Patient 6 | Totals |
| Is patient over 65? | | | | | | | |
| Has patient got more than one other health problem? | | | | | | | |
| Has patient had a fracture in the last year? | | | | | | | |
| Has patient had the pressure sore for more than 3 months? | | | | | | | |
| In which care setting did the pressure sore start? | | | | | | | |
| Does the patient live on his/her own or with an elderly carer? | | | | | | | |

## FEEDBACK

This activity is likely to have reinforced what the text has told you. You may not have identified patients with fractures, although this will depend on your work area, but it is highly likely that many of your patients are over 65 with more than one other health factor to consider. An exception to this would be staff working in young disabled units. It is also likely that several patients may have had their pressure sores for some time, particularly in the community setting. Where the pressure sores started will depend on your work area: if you work on an orthopaedic ward with a high proportion of elderly patients, you may find that several of the sores started with you; if in the community, sores may have started there or been transferred from hospital. You may have been able to pick up patterns from your results, which as the text continues may give you some ideas of particular problems and how you can start to address them.

### Self-assessment   10 MINUTES

1. In David's research (1983), what percentage of patients with sores were over 65?
2. What percentage of over-75-year-olds did Harding et al (1993) find to have long-standing illnesses?
3. Over the next 50 years, which two groups of people are expected to increase in total numbers the most?

## FEEDBACK

1. 85% of the patients with sores were over 65.
2. 70% of the over-75 age group had long-standing illness.
3. The two groups expected to increase are the over-65s and over-85s.

## 1.3 THE ROLE OF SPECIALIST SOCIETIES IN THE SUBJECT OF PRESSURE SORES

As the interest in pressure sores and chronic wounds increased it became apparent that there were individuals who had a specific interest in the subject, and that much work was needed to tackle the problem.

Additionally, people were beginning to look at the same areas of practice, but without liaison with those doing the same thing elsewhere, resulting in duplication of work. As a result several different groups arose, but the one thing that they have in common is increasing knowledge and providing education on tissue viability issues.

### The Tissue Viability Society: TVS

This was one of the first societies to emerge and was open to any person 'concerned, interested or engaged in tissue viability, or the objectives of the society'. Its revised constitution in 1991 gave the objective 'to promote learning and advance education in the study of tissue viability and do all such things as may be conducive to improve techniques for maintaining tissue viability.' Apart from day-to-day running, and being available to give advice to anyone who sought it, their main undertakings which benefit all staff are:

- a magazine entitled *Journal of Tissue Viability*, which was one of the first to cover this subject inclusively in the UK
- two meetings a year which are themed to cover specific issues, e.g. wounds of the lower leg, tissue viability in people with physical disability
- study days on prevention and assessment of pressure sores and more recently leg ulcers, where hospitals can book the session and the society will arrange to come to that venue and hold the sessions.

### The Wound Care Society: WCS

This group was formed in 1987 by a group of nurses who 'were concerned that nursing practice should reflect the progress that has taken place both in theoretical wound healing research and in the developments of new wound care products'. The first year it received sponsorship to get started, after which it was able to function on its own. Again, advice is always available for nursing staff who contact committee members. The aims are:

- to develop a network of nurses with expertise in wound care
- to improve the education of nurses by providing a sound research-based knowledge of wound care
- to disseminate this information to relevant health care workers
- to coordinate information concerning wound care and the treatments available
- to create a platform for the study and discussion of wound care
- to liaise with similar organisations, the ultimate aim being to form an international federation of wound care.

Other initiatives include:

- conferences for trained and student nurse members
- regular supplement in the *Nursing Times* magazine (*Journal of Wound Care Nursing*) on matters relating to wound care. These are sent to members once a year to provide a useful source of information.

## European Wound Management Association: EWMA

This was established following a multidisciplinary conference in 1991 which included delegates from 26 countries. The aim of this group was to 'complement existing societies, and ensure a vehicle for both clinical and scientific issues in wound healing and wound care to be addressed by a multi-disciplinary audience.' (Harding 1992). Membership is multi-disciplinary and world-wide. For staff in general they hold an annual conference in a European country, in which speakers from around the world take part, and a book of the proceedings and presentations is produced after each conference.

## National Association of Tissue Viability Nurses: NATVN

This group was started by a small enthusiastic group of specialist nurses, who felt that they needed support for the often isolated role of nurse specialist. Initially, because of the small number of nurse specialists, making progress was difficult. However, there are now many more tissue viability nurses, and local groups have been formed in the following regions of the UK:

- South West
- North West
- South
- North East
- Midlands
- Scotland.

From these local groups, membership of the NATVN is made up of one representative from each local group. A new constitution is being drawn up. The group intends to look at relevant issues in tissue viability and particularly in relation to the role of the nurse specialist. Each local group tends to have its own focus which is then shared with the main group at the annual meetings, or through their representative on the committee.

Examples are:

- setting up an education course aimed at the needs of the tissue viability nurse specialist
- producing a generic job description to cover the broad outline of the job
- stating what requirements are needed from a pressure-relieving mattress from the user's point of view
- looking at the problems of restrictions of wound dressings in the community.

With commercial companies and individual trusts running their own study days on tissue viability, there is a danger of overload, but at the moment there still seems to be a large audience for any days relating to these issues. Problems arise at the more advanced level, where information begins to seem the same at some of the conferences; however, it cannot be said that there is not a group to suit every sort of member. A welcome addition to the information sources has been the *Journal of Wound Care*, produced 10 times a year, which contains useful articles on many aspects of wound care, and is frequently referenced in this pack. It is also unusual in that it is one of the few commercially produced magazines read and contributed to by different professional groups.

---

**Activity**      **1** HOUR

1. Ask three of your colleagues whether they belong to any of the societies mentioned above. If you have people who belong to different ones, you may be able to pool the information and magazines to the benefit of you all. If not, you may like to think of each joining one.

2. Try to obtain one copy of each magazine or supplement mentioned, and see which one you feel is most useful to you:

   - *Journal of Tissue Viability*
   - *Journal of Wound Care Nursing*
   - *Journal of Wound Care.*

Note: This activity may require longer than 1 hour, depending on the accessibility of magazines.

---

As well as the groups quoted here, many areas have small interested groups, and many of the medical, nursing and paramedic magazines contain articles on tissue viability subjects. It is therefore difficult for anyone to continue to claim ignorance of the subject.

## SUMMARY

In this section you have learned that:

- until recently management of wounds and pressure sores was not based on research-based evidence

- demographic changes mean that the potential is there for the pressure sore problem to get worse, not better

- different specialist societies and journals exist to provide expert education and knowledge for health professionals.

## REFERENCES

Anthony D 1987 Are you in the dark? Nursing Times 83: 25–30

Bennett G, Moody M 1995 Wound care for health professionals. Chapman & Hall, London

Caldock K 1993 The Community White Paper—a nursing perspective. British Journal of Nursing 2(11): 592–597

Charcot J M 1877 On diseases of the nervous system. New Sydenham Society

Clarke M 1988 The nursing prevention of pressure sores in hospital and community patients. Journal of Advanced Nursing 13(3): 365–373

Collier M 1995 Pressure sore development and prevention. Educational leaflet No 3, Vol 1 (revised). Wound Care Society

David J et al 1983 An investigation of the care of patients with established pressure sores. Northwich Park Research Unit, Middlesex

Department of Health 1990 Community care in the next decade and beyond: policy guidelines. HMSO London

Gould D 1985 Pressure for change. Nursing Mirror 161: 28–30

Harding K 1992 Preface. In: Harding K, Leaper D L, Turner T (eds) First European Conference in Advances in Wound Management. Macmillan Magazines, London

Harding K, Jones V, Sinclair A J 1993 Wound care in an ageing population, Journal of Wound Care 2(6): 366–369

Knight B 1985 The history of wound treatments. In Westaby S (ed) Wound care. Heinemann Medical Books, London

Norton D, McLaren R, Exton-Smith A N 1962 An investigation of geriatric nursing problems in hospital. National Corporation for the Care of Old People, London

Oliver E 1994 Maintaining nutritional support in the community. Journal of Tissue Viability 4(1): 28–34

Pajk M, Craven G A, Cameron-Barry J, Shipps T, Bennum N W 1986 Investigating the problem of pressure sores. Journal of Gerontological Nursing 12(7):11–16

Rough M 1994 Pressure sore prevention. Community Outlook (Dec): 32–36

Thompson Rowling J 1961 Pathological changes in mummies. Proceedings of the Royal Society of Medicine 54: 409

Versluysen M 1985 Pressure sores in elderly patients—the epidemiology related to hip operations. Journal of Bone and Joint Surgery 67b(1): 10–13

Versluysen M 1986 How elderly patients with femur fractures develop pressure sores in hospital. British Medical Journal 292(17 May): 1311–1313

Walsh M, Ford P 1989 Nursing rituals—research and rational actions. Heinemann Nursing, Oxford

Winter G 1962 Formation of the scab and the rate of epithelialisation of superficial wounds in the skin of the domestic pig. Nature (193): 293

# The size of the problem

Despite the fact that pressure sores have been around for so long there is still confusion about how to measure the size of the problem, and indeed what to measure. Increasing awareness of the costs involved in pressure sore treatments has raised the profile of the whole subject at government level.

## LEARNING OUTCOMES

At the end of this section you should be aware of:

- how to grade pressure sores
- the different ways to measure the size of the pressure sore problem
- factors affecting data collection
- cost implications of pressure sores for the patients and the NHS.

'The Health of the Nation' discussion paper (DoH 1992) gives targets that the Government hopes to see achieved in relation to a reduction in the number of pressure sores occurring. This has raised the whole profile of the pressure sore problem in all health care settings, and has made it necessary for all areas to start counting pressure sores and to identify in which care setting they started.

Definitions of terms to help you with this whole section are given in Box 2.1.

---

**Box 2.1** Definitions

**Point prevalence:** Snapshot of a defined population with an identified problem at at specific point in time.

**Period prevalence:** Total number of people with an identified problem or condition over a defined period of time.

**Incidence:** Number of people developing a specific condition over a period of time within a defined patient group.

---

## 2.1 GRADING OF PRESSURE SORES

To measure the pressure sore problem it is necessary to have a way of describing sores by their severity and depth. This is particularly important as it is the deep sores which cause the most problems in terms of money and patient suffering. This is why setting targets for reduction in numbers may not be the correct strategy. Evidence of greater awareness will show an increase in the reporting of the less severely graded sores, as nurses recognise the importance of these. Recognising these less severe sores and taking preventive action should reduce the total number of deep sores. The deep sores are expensive in both monetary and human terms, as will be shown later in this section. Several grading systems exist which attempt to describe sores by depth and severity.

### Tissue type

As well as depth of sores, the type of tissue varies. Pressure sores are areas of tissue that have died from lack of oxygen and nutrients, and this results in slough or necrotic tissue. Removal of this tissue is essential both to discover the true depth of the sore and to promote wound healing. There may be tendons, bone or a sinus visible at the base of the sore, once the dead tissue is removed.

As pressure sores begin to heal, healthy granulation tissue will be seen. Sometimes different stages of the healing process can be observed within a single wound; Section 5 will cover this in more detail. As will be seen from the grading systems shown here, some describe the depth only, while others categorise the type of tissue within the wound. As well as grading wounds it is necessary to measure them so that an accurate evaluation of progress can be made in the nursing care plan.

### Systems in common use

It is unfortunate that because for many years pressure sores were not given a high priority people involved in trying to measure and solve the pressure sore problem began to develop their own tools to describe the severity of pressure sores. Whilst this in itself is admirable, it has led to several different grading systems existing with anything from four to six basic categories and some with further sub-categories. Further adaptations have been made by some local health authorities. Three grading systems are shown in this section; they are the Torrance (Table 2.1), Surrey (Table 2.2) and Stirling (Table 2.3) systems. Not all grading systems include damage which occurs at the early stage of pressure sore development, where non-blanching hyperaemia is present.

Non-blanching hyperaemia is an early test for pressure sore damage and is shown by depressing a red area of tissue from which pressure has been removed. If the skin remains red instead of blanching to the touch, this indicates that tissue damage has already occurred and preventive action needs to be instigated. This needs to be started immediately to prevent further tissue breakdown. The physiological reasons for this are considered in Section 3. The fact that not all grading systems include this category shows that the importance of recognising this early-stage pressure damage has not always been recognised. Other stages of pressure damage are: partial skin loss; full thickness skin loss; and full thickness skin loss extending into underlying tissue.

**Table 2.1** Torrance grading system (Torrance 1983)

| Grade | Description |
| --- | --- |
| Stage 1 | Blanching hyperaemia |
| Stage 2 | Non-blanching hyperaemia |
| Stage 3 | Ulceration progresses through the dermis only |
| Stage 4 | The lesion extends into the subcutaneous fat |
| Stage 5 | Infective necrosis penetrates the deep fascia |

**Table 2.2** Surrey grading system (David et al 1983)

| Grade | Description |
| --- | --- |
| Stage 1 | Non-blanching erythema |
| Stage 2 | Superficial break in skin |
| Stage 3 | Destruction of skin without cavity |
| Stage 4 | Destruction of skin with cavity |

**Table 2.3** Stirling grading system (Reid & Morison 1984)

| Stage | Description |
| --- | --- |
| | No clinical evidence of a pressure sore: |
| 0.0 | Normal appearance, intact skin |
| 0.1 | Healed with scarring |
| 0.2 | Tissue damaged but not assessed as a pressure sore |
| | Discoloration of intact skin: |
| 1.1 | Non-blanchable erythema with increased localised heat |
| 1.2 | Blue/purple/black discoloration |
| | Partial thickness skin loss involving epidermis and/or dermis: |
| 2.1 | Blister |
| 2.2 | Abrasion |
| 2.3 | Shallow ulcer without undermining of adjacent tissue |
| 2.4 | Any of these with blue/purple/black discoloration or induration |
| | Full thickness skin loss involving damage or necrosis to subcutaneous tissue but not extending to underlying bone, tendon or joint capsule: |
| 3.1 | Crater, without undermining of adjacent tissue |
| 3.2 | Crater, with undermining of adjacent tissue |
| 3.3 | Sinus, the full extent of which is uncertain |
| 3.4 | Full thickness skin loss, but wound bed is covered with necrotic tissue which masks the true extent of tissue damage |
| | Full thickness skin loss with extensive destruction and tissue necrosis extending to underlying bone, tendon, or joint capsule: |
| 4.1 | Visible exposure of bone, tendon or capsule |
| 4.2 | Sinus assessed as extending to bone, tendon or capsule |

Recognition of pressure damage at an early stage by all staff is the key to an effective prevention strategy, so encouraging staff to report it will raise awareness (Hitch 1995). It will also increase the overall prevalence and incidence of sores for that reporting area, in comparison with areas which only report damage from broken skin upwards, as has been shown in Reader Article 1 (O'Dea 1993). The condition of the surrounding skin should also be noted, as this may indicate an extension of the pressure damage occurring, or damage from another source such as incontinence. When assessing skin that is non-white, relying on visual signs may not be enough (Baxter 1993). The nurse should listen to the patient who may complain of irritation or discomfort. Thickening may be felt at the site of the damage.

## Using grading tools

A major problem with grading tools can be the varying interpretation by different staff even when using the same grading system. This likelihood increases the more complex the system and the more choices that people are given, such as in the systems with several sub-sections to each grading. A recent survey by Healey (1995) showed that none of the three tools mentioned here demonstrated great reliability, especially with the less severe grades of sore, and that the one with the most categories was the least reliable in terms of nurses reporting accurately. Also, sores with mixed tissue type may be difficult to categorise.

**Activity**                    45 MINUTES

Look at Plates 1 and 2 (between pp. 22 and 23).

1. Describe the depth and tissue type of each sore.
2. Using the three grading systems shown, grade both sores using each system.
3. Ask a colleague to carry out the same exercise. Note whether you agree or disagree on your description/grading, and whether you found it easier with one tool rather than another to grade the sores.
4. Repeat this exercise on two patients in your caseload.

## FEEDBACK

### Plate 1

1. You should have described Plate 1 as destruction of the skin without a visible cavity but with discolouration of the area.

2. You should have graded this sore as follows:

    Torrance    3
    Stirling    2.4
    Surrey      3

### Plate 2

1. You should have described this as a mixed sore of full thickness and tissue loss. There is a surrounding margin of granulating tissue with a necrotic area in the centre. When the necrotic tissue was removed from this patient, bone was visible underneath.
2. You should have graded this photo as follows:

    Torrance    5
    Stirling    3.4
    Surrey      4

Did you and your colleague agree or disagree on your gradings? Did you find some grading scores more difficult to use than others, or did they provide more areas for disagreement/discussion? Depending on your results you may have formed some ideas of your own on how user-friendly and/or accurate different systems can be.

## Implications of using grading tools

There have been suggestions for bringing in a national grading system. The reality of this, however, is that areas already using systems may not want to undertake re-education of all staff and risk confusion in grading. Also, if they are recording incidence of pressure sores, this could change their figures if the pressure sore grading system were different, and render their baseline figures meaningless.

This would occur if, for instance, an area had previously not included non-blanching hyperaemia in their figures, and then suddenly introduced this usually large patient group as having pressure damage. Equally, it could be argued that an area reporting non-blanching hyperaemia could overnight achieve their 5–10% (DoH 1992) reduction by excluding these from the data in future reports.

What is obvious is that to measure prevalence and incidence, a grading system should be in place. This should be user-friendly, and all staff should be expected to use it and educated in its use. Grading of sores provides a measurement against which the effectiveness of any care programmes being implemented can be evaluated, in terms of:

- use of pressure relieving equipment
- measures to improve physiological status
- use of a specific wound care product.

These measures correctly used and in conjunction with holistic care will, it is hoped, cause the sore to decrease in depth and size.

Use of the same system across a whole area, including community, private sector and acute care, provides a universal language which will assist in smooth transfer of patients and continuation of appropriate care interventions.

**Activity**                              5 MINUTES

List the advantages of having a grading system in use.

# FEEDBACK

You should have said that the advantages are:

1. to measure sores by severity
2. to help evaluate the effectiveness of care and treatment strategies in use
3. to assist in patient transfer and continuation of care from one care setting to another.

**Self-assessment**                       5 MINUTES

What are four depth categories that can be used to classify pressure sores?

# FEEDBACK

You should have remembered that they are non-blanching hyperaemia (not included in all scales), partial thickness skin loss, full thickness skin loss, and full thickness skin loss extending into underlying tissue.

## 2.2 DATA COLLECTION

While some areas already have monitoring systems in place to measure the size of the problem, others have had to start them up, and there are several factors to consider in relation to obtaining accurate data (see below). Education and staff training in data collection are also needed. It is important too that staff are aware of why data is being collected, and that they receive regular feedback. If this does not occur, they are liable to lose motivation and send in incomplete returns, or

none at all. Accurate baselines need to be established to provide evidence of reduction.

There are two main problem areas related to data collection.

- Accuracy of data provided during the collection period. All patients need to be examined by staff undertaking the survey, as relying on verbal reports from patients or staff in the area is to introduce an element of unreliability.
- Varying methods of collection, particularly relating to grades of pressure sores included in the survey, which can vary from place to place.

There are also ethical and time implications for a prevalence survey covering a large area, especially if the people carrying out the survey do not work there. Incidence data should be recorded by a member of the staff identifying the damage as soon as it occurs, but in the author's experience this is often done retrospectively once a week by a designated person. In acute areas with a high patient turnover, this may result in some patients being excluded from the data.

A further consideration is that until staff start to follow patient episodes instead of targeting areas, inaccurate information will inevitably be provided. An example of this would be a patient developing a pressure sore on a ward, which would be recorded as starting in the hospital. The patient is then transferred to the community, where the district nurse records the sore as being present on admission to her caseload, and originating in the hospital. A week later the patient is admitted to a different ward with a chest infection, where the staff record that he has a pressure sore which started in the community. This is incorrect. Again, this is where accurate transfer information between staff and computerisation across all health care settings would begin to provide the true picture of where pressure sores start, where they improve, and where they deteriorate.

To be able to see whether government targets are being achieved, it is necessary to understand how to measure the size of the pressure sore problem and to appreciate any potential problems with data collection which may affect the results. Simply counting the numbers of sores present will not provide all the information required.

### Measuring the size of the pressure sore problem

Measuring the size of the pressure sore problem is a difficult exercise, made worse by lack of uniformity in:

- grading of sores
- monitoring tools
- different populations being studied.

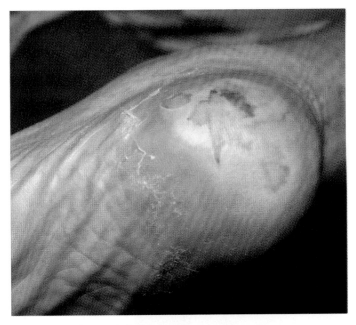

**Plate 1** *(See Section 2, Activity, p. 21.)*

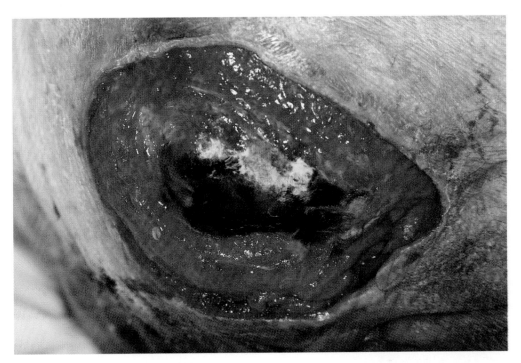

**Plate 2** *(See Section 2, Activity, p. 21.)*

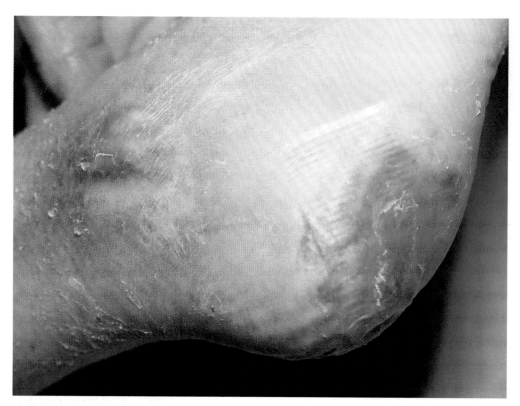

**Plate 3** Non-blanching hyperaemia.

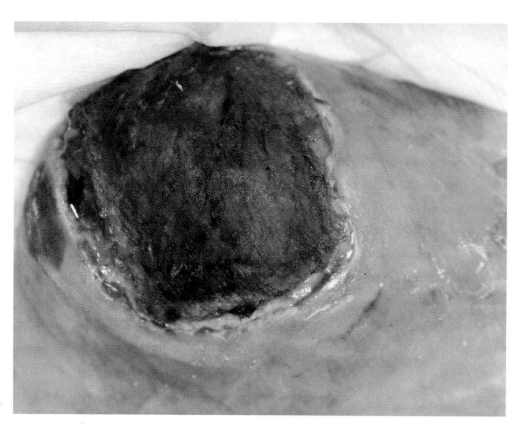

**Plate 4** Pressure sore on heel showing black, leathery appearance following skin breakdown.

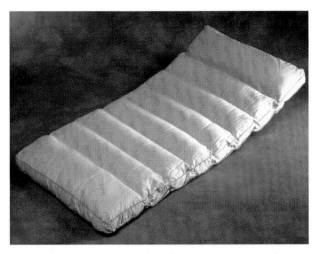

**Plate 5** Fibre-filled overlay (courtesy of HNE, Luton).

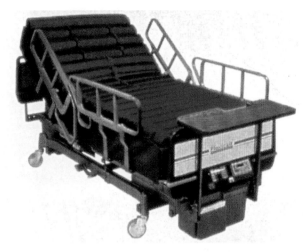

**Plate 7** Low air loss bed (courtesy of Support Systems International, Leicester).

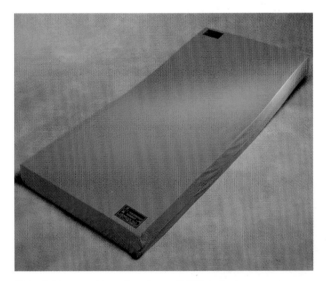

**Plate 6** Foam mattress (courtesy of HNE, Luton).

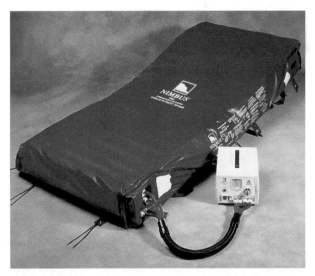

**Plate 8** Mattress replacement (courtesy of HNE, Luton).

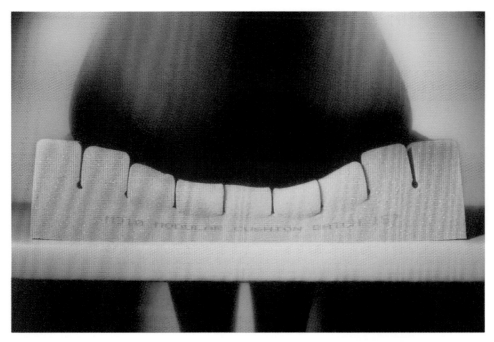

**Plate 9** Foam pressure-reducing cushion (courtesy of Medical Support Systems, Cardiff).

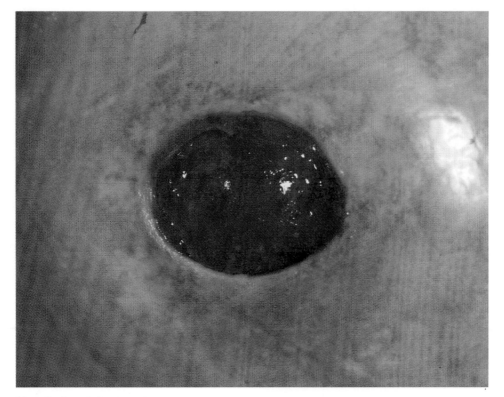

**Plate 10** Granulating wound.

Government targets have raised the whole profile, with the result that purchasers are wanting to know where and why their patients develop pressure sores, and providers are finding their figures used as quality indicators.

In order to comply with government targets, the 'Health of the Nation' document (DoH 1992) states that 'the first task for health authorities would be to establish the baseline incidence and prevalence of the condition'.

How people measure and report sores will also affect results and comparisons, although most comparisons should not be carried out unless the patient populations and reporting methods are the same. There are two accepted ways of measuring pressure sores—prevalence and incidence—and each gives different results.

## Prevalence

There are two different types of prevalence:

- point prevalence
- period prevalence.

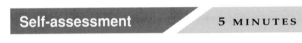

Can you remember the difference between point prevalence and period prevalence? Write down the definitions.

● ● ● ● ● ● ● ● ● ● ● ● ● ● ● ● ● ● ● ● ● ● ● ● ● ● ● ● ● ● ● ●

## FEEDBACK

You should have said that point prevalence is a snapshot of a defined population with an identified problem at a specific point in time, while period prevalence is the total number of people with an identified problem or condition over a defined period of time. In other words, a survey of all patients in a care setting on 1 day will give a point prevalence for that day. A count of all patients with a pressure sore in a care setting over 1 week will give a period prevalence for 1 week. In these surveys the interest is in the total number of patients with pressure sores, regardless of where they started.

● ● ● ● ● ● ● ● ● ● ● ● ● ● ● ● ● ● ● ● ● ● ● ● ● ● ● ● ● ● ● ●

The most commonly acquired prevalence figures are from a point prevalence survey carried out over 1 day and recording every patient in the chosen care setting who has a pressure sore. To obtain the point prevalence as a percentage, it is necessary to know the total number of patients in the area on that day.

Thus:

$$\text{Prevalence} = \frac{\text{patients with damage} \times 100}{\text{total population}}$$

**Example.** 6 patients with pressure damage in a ward of 24 patients would give a prevalence of 25%: $6 \times 100 \div 24 = 25$. This can be applied to small areas such as a ward or caseload, or to whole populations such as hospitals.

## Incidence

Incidence of pressure sores may prove more useful as a quality indicator because of the type of information it provides. It tells you how many patients have developed a pressure sore while in a particular care setting over a defined time.

Incidence allows you to study any size of population over a chosen time span which can be as little as 1 week or up to 1 year or more. Working out the percentage again requires the total number of patients cared for in the chosen care setting over the specified time.

**Example.** To calculate the incidence of pressure sores in a district nurse caseload during a 1-month period, you need the following information:

Total caseload = 90 patients

Number of patients developing sores at home this month = 2

$$\text{Incidence} = 2 \times 100 \div 90 = 2\%$$
(to nearest decimal point)

If incidence within a unit or hospital is being measured, care needs to be taken not to duplicate data. This can occur when a patient is recorded by a ward as having developed pressure damage, and is then transferred to another ward who also record the damage as being hospital acquired on the previous ward. This is an argument for computerised systems which will recognise when this has happened.

Incidence also enables staff to identify problems which may be preventable in their own areas. A critical look at the care planning and resources provided may highlight improvements in care which might have prevented development of a pressure sore.

Estimates of both prevalence and incidence are affected by the number of patients in a care setting who are at risk of developing a condition, in this case pressure sores. Patients whose illness or condition makes them more susceptible to pressure damage are in a higher-risk group and will have a higher incidence of pressure sores unless more resources are used. Resources means anything from more equipment, to more staff, to providing educational input, depending on the need of that particular area.

## Activity                    1½–2 HOURS

Having obtained the permission of your manager, complete the following activity. Take either 1 day or 1 week, and count up all the patients you see in your caseload or ward with pressure damage.

1. State whether you have obtained a point prevalence or period prevalence or incidence rate for your area.

2. Grade the pressure sores and, using Table 2.4:
   a. Note where on the body the pressure sores occur, entering the grade in the appropriate column. You may find that some patients have more than one pressure sore to record.
   b. Under the source column write in where the sore started, e.g. home, hospital, nursing home.

Can you identify any other information which this exercise has provided you with which can be used as quality indicators of care?

● ● ● ● ● ● ● ● ● ● ● ● ● ● ● ● ● ● ● ● ● ● ● ● ● ● ● ● ● ●

## FEEDBACK

You should have answered Question 1 as follows. A survey carried out on 1 day will have provided a point prevalence, a survey over 1 week a period prevalence.

Your completed table should enable you to see:

- which grade of sores started in your own area.
- which body sites are most affected. This may highlight problems for you to look at, for instance if you have a number of heel sores which have started in your area, can you identify why?

You may have identified a high number of sores coming into your area from another care setting, suggesting the need for liaison with that area. You may not have been able to identify the source of the sore from your notes and this may have implications, particularly if a complaint is registered regarding care to the patient and the fact that he or she has developed a pressure sore.

● ● ● ● ● ● ● ● ● ● ● ● ● ● ● ● ● ● ● ● ● ● ● ● ● ● ● ● ● ● ● ●

This activity should have made you realise that collecting specific data can also provide you with further useful information and many surveys now incorporate information such as:

- identifying patients at risk
- equipment in use
- involvement of other health care professionals etc.

All of these can be linked to the quality of care provided. This baseline information makes it possible to monitor the effectiveness of a prevention programme once implemented. This is the correct way to use the data provided, to help staff improve and monitor the quality of care relating to pressure sores in their own areas, rather than providing potentially irrelevant comparisons between different patient populations.

## Self-assessment                10 MINUTES

Which measurement provides a better quality indicator of care for a specific area, prevalence or incidence? Give a reason for your answer.

| Table 2.4 | | | | | | | |
| --- | --- | --- | --- | --- | --- | --- | --- |
| Patient | Source | Sacrum | Heels | Hips | Buttocks | Elbows | Other (specify) |
| 1 | | | | | | | |
| 2 | | | | | | | |
| 3 | | | | | | | |
| 4 | | | | | | | |
| 5 | | | | | | | |
| 6 | | | | | | | |
| Rule up another sheet if you have more than six patients to record. | | | | | | | |

## FEEDBACK

Incidence identifies patients in your own group who have developed pressure sores, thus providing an opportunity for staff to look at the care being provided and identify any problems. Prevalence only tells you how many patients in total have pressure damage, not how many developed a pressure sore in your area.

## 2.3 THE COST OF PRESSURE SORES

The financial cost of pressure sores has long been hidden, as money spent on expensive treatments for deep sores has either been found from existing budgets, or not found at all. In the latter cases, nursing staff cope with these large wounds as best they can. The Patients' Charter and increasing awareness of the problem have finally raised this item at managerial level.

There can be little doubt that increasing interest at national and regional level in the problem of pressure sores is cost driven. Cost can be divided into two categories:

- financial costs
- quality of life costs to patients and carers.

### Financial costs

The recently produced guide for purchasers and providers (DoH 1993) is one of the first major documents to make the point that prevention may cost as much as treatment. Cullum & Shakespeare (1994), in their review of this document and the report on which it is based, raise the issue that a logical interpretation might be that it is not worth paying out for prevention and better to accept the inevitable treatment costs.

They do, however, list some factors which should underpin a prevention strategy and stress that these must be seen to be as cost effective as can be shown by data collection, particularly if a decrease in patients developing deep sores can be shown. Similarly, Bridel (1995) quotes incidence studies which show that the majority of pressure sores, 95%, are in the superficial group. She asks whether attention should be focused on prevention of these superficial sores or treatment of the less common, but extremely expensive, cavity wounds. It could be argued that a percentage of superficial sores progress to become cavity sores, so prevention of superficial sores should be a key target. This does not solve the problem, which will be looked at in the risk assessment section (p. 39), of why some

patients develop deep sores while others do not. Accurate data collection will again show how many superficial sores in a care setting progress to become deep sores.

The biggest ongoing costs are specialised equipment, wound dressings, and nurse time, especially in the community where travel time and costs are included. However, if patients or relatives sue for development of pressure sores, paying out for this can be far more expensive than if money had been invested in a planned strategy of prevention. Grounds for people suing for development of a pressure sore are discussed in Section 6.1.

Litigation costs quoted by Silver (1989) were for £100 000 for a single patient episode. Another cost gaining importance in these days of increased productivity is blocking of an acute bed caused by a patient who develops pressure sores, and this is why many patients who would have previously been kept in hospital for care until their pressure sores were less severe, are now discharged back into the community with cavity wounds.

### Quality of life costs

The suggestion of withholding preventive measures would also be to totally ignore the quality of life issues involved for patients and their carers. Very little has been written on this and yet, with the Patients' Charter and quality care initiatives, this should be of primary concern to all staff involved in looking after patients, especially those recognised as being at high risk of pressure damage.

Price & Harding (1993) look at some of the tools developed which attempt to measure quality of life. The main areas which are covered are:

- psychological aspects such as anxiety or depression
- social aspects, including relationships and home situation
- occupational aspects, or role function in life
- physical aspects, including well-being and general health.

Looking at a patient's quality of life involves seeing how much effect their illness or wound has had on these four areas of their life.

Many patients who develop pressure damage are elderly. Their quality of life may well not be high anyway, and this may be one reason why pressure sores have for so long been given a low priority. Even now, the main reason for raising awareness is because of the financial cost to the NHS. This should not be the case; care strategies should be aimed at protecting from damage those less able to help themselves. Pressure sores also place an increasing burden on carers, who may need to move the patient more frequently, be unable to take the patient out, or have to cope with a patient suffering from depression caused by the pressure sore.

For this activity ask your manager for permission to carry it out, and also check that you do not need ethical clearance to involve the patient. This is not likely as long as you obtain the patient's consent to take part and ensure confidentiality as you will not be altering the patient's treatment in any way. Select a consenting patient in your care who has got or has had a pressure sore of full skin thickness or more. Using the sliding scale in Table 2.5, fill in the column headed 'Nurse' with the numbers that best reflect the effect you think the pressure sore has had on the patient in each of the areas listed. Then explain the scale to the patient and get him or her to do the same. For example, if you think the patient is getting less sleep than usual because of the pressure sore, score 3. Do not ask the patient before filling in your column, the idea being to see if you are aware of problems your patient has in relation to the pressure sore. When both columns have been filled in, compare the two results.

## FEEDBACK

This exercise should raise your awareness of how pressure sores can affect the patient's quality of life.

You may have found that both you and the patient recorded similar scores, or there may have been areas highlighted by the patient's answers which showed effects of which you were unaware. This activity may help you to improve your care planning and awareness of problems for future patients.

List five financial cost factors which can be incurred in pressure sore management.

## FEEDBACK

You should have identified: specialised equipment, wound dressings, nurse time, litigation, and decreased productivity in acute areas from bed blocking.

## Conclusion

The preceding section of this module has shown that pressure sores have been a recognised problem for a considerable time, although the combination of factors contributing to their occurrence has not always been acknowledged. Individuals have developed an interest in the subject and attempted to raise awareness, and any literature review will show a sharp increase in relevant literature since the 1980s.

| Table 2.5 | | |
|---|---|---|
| *Activity* | *Nurse* | *Patient* |
| Social life | | |
| Work | | |
| Mobility | | |
| Sleep | | |
| State of mind | | |
| Appetite | | |
| Relationships | | |
| *Scale* | | |

| 1 | 2 | 3 | 4 | 5 |
|---|---|---|---|---|
| Has had no impact on activity or state of mind | Has had a little impact on activity or state of mind | Has moderately impacted on activity or state of mind | Has greatly impacted on activity or state of mind | Has had a seriously bad effect on activity or state of mind |

However, not until 1992 did the Department of Health feel it necessary to step in. Their discussion document on 'Health of the Nation' says 'the government view is that an annual reduction of at least 5–10% in their incidence would be a reasonable target' (DoH 1992). In the same document, they quote a prevalence rate of hospital patients as 6.7%, but the work reported by O'Dea (1993) (see Reader Article 1) found an overall prevalence in hospitals of 18.6%, or 10.1% excluding non-blanching hyperaemia.

Although the goal for a reduction in pressure sores is not one of the key target areas in the 'Health of the Nation' document, it has been taken on board by many purchasers who now want figures relating to the size of the problem from their providers. However, not taken into account by all areas is that incidence and prevalence figures also relate to the number of patients at risk, and target setting should relate to this and vary according to the local population (Shakespeare 1994).

## Activity                                5 MINUTES

Article 1 in the Reader provides a comprehensive look at the process of monitoring prevalence, and although the work has been done in the acute setting, it contains interesting information for all nurses. Look through this article again and note down the average percentage of patients quoted as developing pressure sores in hospital.

## FEEDBACK

You should have said that an average of 68.2% of patients who develop pressure sores develop them in hospital.

## Self-assessment                         10 MINUTES

1. What is the government target for annual reduction in hospital pressure sore incidence?

2. Which of the following figures—5.2%, 6.7%, 10.1%, 12.2%, 16.1%, 18.6%—does:

   a. the 'Health of the Nation' document quote as prevalence of pressure sores in hospitals in the UK?

   b. O'Dea suggest is a more realistic overall hospital prevalence rate?

## FEEDBACK

You should have said:

1. The government target for reduction in pressure sore incidence is 5–10%.

2. a. The 'Health of the Nation' document sets the prevalence rates in hospitals in the UK as 6.7%.

   b. O'Dea suggests that a more realistic overall hospital prevalence is 18.6%.

## SUMMARY

This section should have shown you that:

- lack of national monitoring and grading scales causes problems with data collection

- there is a difference between measuring prevalence and incidence

- government targets for reduction may be affected by methods of data collection

- pressure sores are expensive in both monetary and quality of life costs.

REFERENCES

Baxter C 1993 Observing skin. Community Outlook (Jan): 21–22
Bridel J 1995 The epidemiology of pressure sores. In: The Ten Percent Challenge Conference. Pegasus Airwave, England
Cullum N, Shakespeare P 1994 Pressure sores, a key quality indicator. Journal of Tissue Viability 1.4(2): 60–62
David J A, Chapman R G, Chapman E J et al 1983 An investigation of the current methods used in nursing for care of patients with established pressure sores. Nursing Practice Research Unit, Harrow
Department of Health 1992 The health of the nation. HMSO, London
Department of Health 1993 Pressure sores—a key quality indicator. DoH, Lancashire
Healey F 1995 The reliability and utility of pressure sore grading scales. Journal of Tissue Viability 5(4): 111–114
Hitch S 1995 NHS Executive Nursing Directorate, strategy for major clinical guidelines, prevention and management of pressure sores a literature review. Journal of Tissue Viability 5(1): 3–11
Price D, Harding K 1993 Defining quality of life. Journal of Wound Care 2(5): 304–307
Reid J, Morison M J 1994 Towards consensus, classification of pressure sores. Journal of Wound Care 3(3): 157–160
Shakespeare P 1994 Scoring the risk scores. Journal of Tissue Viability 4(1): 21–22
Silver J 1989 Editorial. Care, Science and Practice (March): 2
Torrance C 1983 Pressure sores, aetiology, treatment and prevention. Croom Helm, London

# 3 Causes of pressure sores

There are many suspected causes of pressure sores. The main cause is pressure, but the effects of this are increased by forces which cause distortion to the tissues. Additionally there are many other factors relating to external influences, such as how or where the patients are positioned, and physiological factors which play a part in pressure sore development. In an attempt to recognise patients who are at an increased risk of pressure sore development, tools have been developed which are used to assess patients in relation to how many risk factors they are exposed to. This section will look in detail at these causes or risk factors and the use of risk assessment tools.

## LEARNING OUTCOMES

At the end of this section you should be able to:

- describe the relevant physiology and pathophysiology relating to pressure sore development
- name the potential risk factors for pressure sore development, and the two main groups in which they occur
- list the factors which can contribute to a poor nutritional intake for patients in different care settings
- name four risk assessment tools and identify the advantages and drawbacks of using these as indicators of patients who will develop pressure sores.

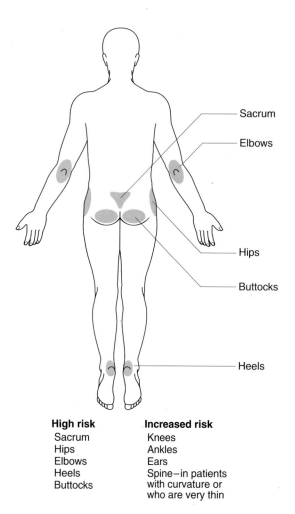

| High risk | Increased risk |
|---|---|
| Sacrum | Knees |
| Hips | Ankles |
| Elbows | Ears |
| Heels | Spine – in patients |
| Buttocks | with curvature or |
| | who are very thin |

**Fig. 3.1** Examples of common pressure sore sites.

## 3.1 ANATOMY AND PHYSIOLOGY

Any nurse involved in pressure sore prevention and management will know that certain parts of the body are more susceptible to damage than others. These areas, typically bony prominences, are exposed to increased pressure loading. See Figure 3.1 for an illustration of the most common sites.

Pressure sores form as a result of damage to the skin and its vascular supply, which, if the pressure is left unrelieved, will cause damage through the full depth of tissues to the bone. To understand the causes of pressure sores, it is necessary to have a working knowledge of the skin and its vascular supply.

Skin is the biggest organ of the body and comprises two main layers, the epidermis and the dermis (Fig. 3.2). It is a dynamic structure in which cell replacement and modification in response to local need is a continual process through life (Barton & Barton 1981). There is a subdermal layer of fat in which blood vessels and nerves lie and also the sweat glands and hair follicles originate. The main functions of skin are:

- temperature regulation
- sensory perception
- excretion of waste
- protection from mechanical, physical and bacterial damage.

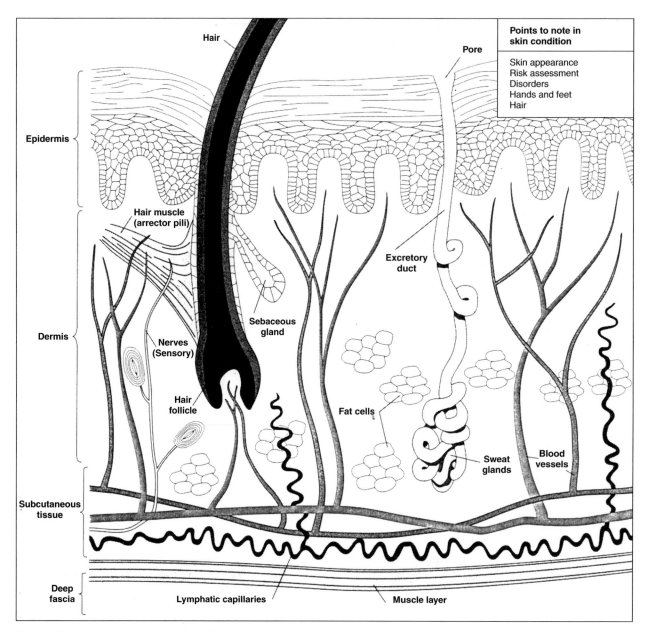

**Fig. 3.2** Cross-section of skin (reproduced from Collier 1994 by kind permission).

## Epidermis

This is the top covering layer and four main types of cells can be found here:

- keratinocytes—the main cells; they help to make skin waterproof by secretion of glycolipid
- melanocytes—which contain pigment to give us our skin colouring, and are affected by genetic make-up, environment and hormones
- Langerhans cells—which form part of the immune system, are derived from bone marrow, and are constantly being renewed
- Merkel cells—which allow for sensation of touch.

## Dermis

This is the second layer down and its main contents are collagen and elastin fibres, providing tensile strength. The blood vessels, nerves, glands and hair follicles also originate here (see Fig. 3.2). There are two layers in the dermis, which are:

1. The papillary layer, which is the smaller layer and provides mechanical anchorage, metabolic support and cell maintenance, and consists of papillae with capillary loops.
2. The reticular layer, attached to underlying structures, bones etc., by the subcutaneous layer. In this layer are the pacinian corpuscles with

nerve endings sensitive to pressure. The main constituents of this layer are collagen, glands and hair follicles.

## Collagen

Collagen is a framework made up of protein fibres, which are essential for wound repair. The collagen/elastin matrix exists to protect the internal structures of the body and also to protect the interstitial fluid and cell content from external pressure. It achieves this by the action of extension and recoil through rotation and alignment. This means that when external pressure is applied the fibres rotate to approach a parallel alignment instead of maintaining their normal configuration. This provides protection to underlying interstitial fluids and cells by forming a more elastic barrier than normal between the pressure point and the underlying tissue.

The quantity of collagen in the skin is known to be affected by:

- age—this reduces the collagen/elastin matrix because of a slowing down in collagen synthesis
- steroids—these imitate the effect of ageing on the body with the same effect
- nutrients—not completely proven, but assumed to reduce collagen synthesis (Bridel 1993)
- ultraviolet light—this weakens and thins the collagen layer.

All of these reduce the protective function of the collagen/elastin matrix, increasing the susceptibility of the patient to the effects of pressure.

### Activity                                    15 MINUTES

Think of two patients in your caseload with pressure damage, then using the space below, make a list of any of the factors mentioned above which are likely to be contributing to a reduction in the effects of the collagen/elastin matrix.

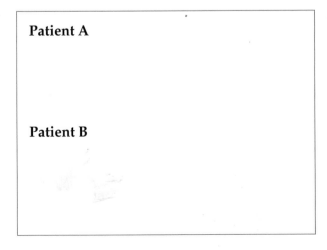

**Patient A**

**Patient B**

## FEEDBACK

You may have a patient who is elderly and on steroids as an example, or one who has all of the risk factors mentioned. The actual causes and their effect will be looked at in more detail later in this section.

## Vascular system

The blood supply to the dermis and epidermis is a complex network of vessels, bringing in the necessary oxygen and nutrients. Capillaries play an essential role, bringing in the blood, allowing exchange of tissue fluids, aiding in temperature regulation and removing waste materials. The blood flow through is not constant, and much tissue fluid exchange occurs when the capillaries are closed, estimated at 60–95% of the time. Capillaries are fragile structures and the mechanism controlling them is sensitive to any changes, particularly occlusion such as can occur from external loading, that is the pressure applied from outside the body. The damage that then occurs to the vascular system is a key component in pressure sore development. See Figure 3.3.

## Nerve endings

Nerve endings are also found in the skin, specifically ones relating to:

- touch
- temperature recognition, hot or cold
- positioning of a limb.

Some areas have more nerve endings than others, e.g. fingertip (touch), tongue (taste).

## Lymphatic system

The main functions of the lymphatic system are:

- Drainage—by taking fluid from the interstitial space and returning it to the circulatory system. Interstitial fluid provides a buffer between the cells.
- Defence—there are numerous lymphatic capillaries in the reticular layer of the skin and defence cells in these recognise foreign cells and set off the body's defence mechanism.

## 3.2 PATHOPHYSIOLOGY

Historically, development of pressure sores was seen solely as an indicator of bad nursing care, with the result that nursing staff feel guilty when pressure sores develop (Benbow 1992). Fortunately, it is now recognised that a variety of factors contribute to pressure damage, although with the exception of immobility and resulting pressure, there is lack of consensus on the relevance of the other frequently quoted causes, as can be seen by the factors included or omitted from the different risk assessment tools shown later in this section. In order to understand how pressure sores develop, it is necessary to study the pathophysiological processes which occur when pressure is applied.

Two processes result in development of pressure sores: 'occlusion of blood vessels by external pressure and endothelial damage of arterioles and the microcirculation due to the application of disruptive and shear forces' (Barton & Barton 1981).

## The effects of pressure

The effect of pressure being applied is occlusion of the blood supply. When the pressure is removed, redness of the skin is visible, caused by the rush of blood back into the tissues. This is known as reactive hyperaemia and is the body's attempt to reduce the oxygen deficiency and remove the waste products which have accumulated as a result of occlusion of the blood vessels. This response indicates that the microcirculation is still intact. If pressure continues unrelieved the next stage is non-blanching hyperaemia, where the redness remains after the load is removed (see Plate 3, between pp. 22 and 23).

The skin itself is better able to withstand pressure and shear forces than the underlying tissues because of its vascularity, so non-blanching hyperaemia indicates that tissue damage has already occurred, and the fingertip test should be used to confirm this. In the fingertip test pressure is applied to the reddened area; if this does not result in the skin blanching or turning white, then tissue damage has begun.

A key to whether permanent tissue damage has occurred is whether the lymphatic system is still functioning. Prolonged pressure will damage lymph vessels and/or affect the level of interstitial fluid, reducing its buffering effect between the cells. Sudden removal of the pressure source reduces the interstitial fluid and can cause the capillaries to burst. The resultant anoxia and waste build-up lead to necrosis or tissue death, shown by discoloration and hard swelling. The discoloration is often purplish in colour progressing to black as total cell death occurs. It is important to be aware that the skin may still be intact at this stage, as extensive underlying damage can occur before the epidermis breaks. This is why discoloured pressure sores often feel soft and spongy when touched. When the skin does break down, exposure to air turns the dead tissue hard, black and leathery (see Plate 4, between pp. 22 and 23).

As non-blanching hyperaemia is the first visible stage of this process, it is essential that all staff learn to recognise it and take immediate action to reverse the process taking place. Figure 3.3 provides a flow chart of these events.

Signs to look for that indicate pressure damage include:

- non-blanching hyperaemia
- swelling, indicating damage to the lymphatic system
- induration/discolouration from tissue damage and cell death
- blistering, indicating damage to the skin.

## Shearing

Shear is a mechanical stress which moves tissues parallel to the surface that the patient is sitting or lying on, causing tearing to take place. An example of this occurs when a patient starts to slide down the bed and the result of this is tearing of the tissues from the structures to which they are attached. This results in damage to the microcirculation especially in the subcutaneous layer. Bridel (1993) reports that this damage activates the clotting mechanism which causes occlusion of the damaged vessels, increasing the risk of necrosis. As well as disrupting underlying tissues, shearing may produce eczema or excoriation of the skin, which can be made worse if the skin is wet from urine or sweat. This break in the skin then breaches the defence mechanism and introduction of bacteria to the tissues can occur resulting in necrosis from sepsis.

| Activity | 40 MINUTES |

Look at Table 3.1. The middle column contains the different stages of tissue breakdown. On the left-hand side, write down the pathophysiological changes that are occurring as each stage is reached. On the right-hand side, write down what can be seen or felt at each stage. The first row is filled in as an example.

## FEEDBACK

Your table entries should be similar to those in Table 3.2. This exercise is to help you know whether you have understood what occurs to start off a pressure sore, and whether you can identify the signs to look for in your own patients.

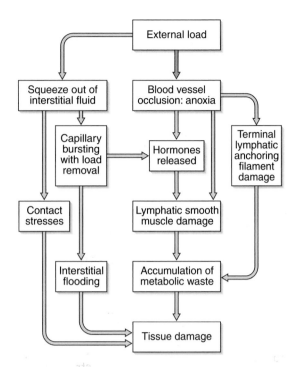

**Fig. 3.3** Proposed mechanism for mechanical-stress-induced tissue necrosis (Krouskop 1983).

### Table 3.1

| Pathophysiological changes | Staging | Visible or felt |
|---|---|---|
| Flush of blood into tissue following removal of pressure | Reactive hyperaemia | Redness which goes away when pressure removed |
|  | Non-blanching hyperaemia |  |
|  | Oedema |  |
|  | Necrosis |  |
|  | Visible ulcer |  |

### Table 3.2  Staging of pressure sores

| Pathophysiological changes | Staging | Visible or felt |
|---|---|---|
| Flush of blood into tissue following removal of pressure | Reactive hyperaemia | Redness which goes away when pressure removed |
| Disruption of the microcirculation | Non-blanching hyperaemia | Redness which stays and does not blanch to the fingertip test |
| Capillaries burst and damage to the lymphatic vessels | Oedema | Swelling |
| Tissue death | Necrosis | Discoloration |
| Continuation of tissue death | Visible ulcer | Appearance of slough, wound soft and spongy |

## 3.3 THE TYPE AND DURATION OF PRESSURE

That pressure is the main causative factor of pressure sores is well known, but of course it is not that simple. Questions that need answering are:

- How much pressure?
- Exerted over how long?
- Affecting what parts of the body?

There is still a lot of work being done on these aspects, and all the answers are not yet available, but it is important to be aware of work done so far on this subject. It may help towards identifying why some patients develop pressure sores while others do not. There are three main types of pressure relative to pressure sores; these are:

- vertical pressure
- tissue interface pressure
- capillary closing pressure.

### Vertical pressure

This is pressure passing straight down from the point of contact to underlying bone, and compressing all the tissues in between. These vary with the sites of sores, but include dermis, muscle, subcutaneous tissue and fat. The greater degree of damage occurs near the bone, which is why by the time damage is visible on the skin, it is often too late to start preventive measures. Barton & Barton (1981) describe this as type 2 pressure damage.

### Tissue interface pressure

This is the pressure 'applied to the epidermis by the surface that is supporting it' (Burman & O'Dea 1994). This is the most commonly measured pressure and is calculated by using the formula:

$$\text{Interface pressure} = \frac{\text{patient weight}}{\text{surface area supported}}$$

There are also gauges which can be placed under patients to measure the pressure, but these vary from simple hand-held instruments measuring one point of contact only, to gauges with several sensors which provide a readout of the pressures at different points on the body. In the past, interface pressures have been quoted in support of purchasing a particular type of mattress, as can be seen by looking at literature used by company representatives; the lower the pressure measurement, the less risk of patients developing pressure damage. This fails to take into account different patient weights which can affect the loading on different mattresses, their

other risk factors, such as poor health, and indeed the more critical figure of capillary closing pressure.

### Capillary closing pressure

This is the pressure at which the capillaries can no longer function, causing collapse and cessation of blood flow. For many years, this figure has been assumed to be in the region of 32 mmHg, based on original work by Landis (1930), but it seems likely that ill and compromised people may develop problems at pressures lower than this. Bridel (1993) discusses some of the pitfalls of relying on this theory alone when looking at causative factors. Capillary closing pressure can only be measured by inserting sensors into the body, and is therefore not a practical measurement in the majority of cases. Nonetheless, it is the more important measurement as regards pressure damage because of the direct effects on the vascular system. It is still affected by other factors, such as:

- amount of fat adjacent to bone
- general state of the vascular system supplying the skin
- physical condition
- systemic blood pressure.

There is also evidence of an autoregulatory mechanism which the capillary network can use to combat certain amounts of pressure (Bridel 1993).

### Shear and friction forces

Shear is a distorting force, and this distortion and the stretching of the skin cause the damage already described in Section 3.2. Typically, shearing forces are applied when patients begin to slide down the bed or off a chair. The tissues begin to move before the bone, and the support surface remains static. This parallel pull causes tearing of the tissues as well as distortion. Often associated with this is friction, which is the rubbing together of two surfaces. Incorrect lifting can produce friction if patients are scraped along the mattress surface, and patients scuffing their heels on the bed is a common cause. Dampness of the skin, as can occur with incontinence, makes this problem worse since it reduces the strength of the skin by causing maceration and rashes (Bergstrom et al 1987).

**Activity**                    10 MINUTES

In the examples given below, identify which type of pressure or force being applied is causing the main risk of developing pressure sores. More than one may apply.

1. Patient lying on an operating table for more than 4 hours.
2. Patient sitting in an armchair and constantly sliding down it.
3. Immobile patient sitting out in a chair all day.

• • • • • • • • • • • • • • • • • • • • • • • • • • • • • • • •

## FEEDBACK

You should have said this.

1. The most important force here is the tissue interface pressure which will be very high, but vertical pressure is also being applied.
2. The most important force here is the shearing occurring from the sliding movement; friction may also play a part, particularly if the patient is drag lifted up the chair by staff.
3. The vertical pressure on this patient will be very high.

You may have identified other pressures, but those listed are the critical ones in these cases. Linking this to what has already been said in Section 3.2, it should now be obvious that patients exposed to pressure and shear combined have the potential for the most serious and deep pressure damage to occur.

• • • • • • • • • • • • • • • • • • • • • • • • • • • • • • • •

Davies (1994) lists different strategies used by nurses to reduce the effects of pressure. These include:

• sheepskins
• barrier creams
• film dressings
• tilting the foot of the bed, to prevent the patient from sliding
• employing correct lifting techniques.

She also highlights the fact that only the factor relating to lifting techniques is supported by evidence as being effective, and points out a need for nursing staff to support their actions scientifically. However, if you employ some of the other methods in your own area, they may help to alleviate the effects of shear and friction as follows.

• Sheepskins do not provide pressure relief, but do reduce a patient's likelihood of sliding down the bed or chair. Any effect they have is greatly reduced once they have been washed a few times.
• Barrier creams can be used to reduce the effects of incontinence on the skin; however, it should be remembered that this does not solve the problem of why the patient is incontinent, and this should be more fully investigated. Since use of creams, powders, etc. on the skin is an extrinsic factor contributing to pressure sores, they should be a last resort.
• Film dressings do reduce friction, but again not pressure, so may lead to a false sense of security if applied to heels. Also they can cause damage to some patients with very thin skin, especially if incorrectly applied and removed. This will be discussed more in the section on wound dressings (p. 78).
• Patients may slide down the bed if they have been incorrectly lifted. A further contributory factor would be incorrect support or positioning of the patient.

This activity may make you rethink some of your ward or caseload management of patients.

In 1959 Kosiak suggested a relationship between the amount and duration of pressure applied in pressure sore development. This is another area of ongoing controversy, and again Bridel (1993) discusses some of the problems relating to this theory. This also goes some way to explaining the different time and pressure measurements used by manufacturers who make alternating pressure relief systems. These systems are explained in Section 4. Bader (1990) suggests that there are two possible reactions to pressure, the first being reactive hyperaemia where the blood returns to the tissues following occlusion bringing with it nutrients and oxygen, and the second, the alternative response, caused by impaired vasomotor control mechanisms, where the return of blood to the tissues would require extended periods of pressure relief, as the body's response slows down because of constant loading. This theory supports the importance of the time factor, but also raises the issue of pressure being constantly applied to the same area of tissue. This may be one reason why some patients still develop pressure sores despite 2-hourly turning.

There is still much work to be done in this area, as all the effects of different types of pressure are not yet fully understood. What is emerging is that repetitive loading may predispose to trauma, and that pressures and shear forces which cause damage to the microcirculation that result in lack of nutrients and oxygen in the tissues are the main physical causes of pressure damage.

| Self-assessment | 45 MINUTES |
|---|---|

1. What are the functions of the skin?
2. What is the effect of ageing on the collagen layer?
3. What is the main function of the collagen/elastin matrix and how does it work?
4. What are the main functions of the capillaries?

5. What are the main functions of the lymphatic system?
6. Suggest two ways in which tissue interface pressure can be measured.
7. Give a definition of capillary closing pressure.

## FEEDBACK

You should have given the following answers.

1. The functions of skin are: temperature regulation, sensory perception, excretion of waste and protection from damage.
2. Ageing reduces collagen synthesis, causing a reduction in the collagen/elastin matrix.
3. The main function of this matrix is to protect the internal structures of the body and the interstitial fluid from external pressures. It does this by buffering the interstitial fluid from external loading, and by responding to external pressure by rotating the fibres, so that they form a parallel alignment, which provides a protective barrier to underlying tissues.
4. Capillaries bring blood to the tissues, allowing exchange of tissue fluid and removing any waste.
5. The main functions of the lymphatic system are defence and to provide a drainage system.
6. Tissue interface pressure can be measured by using the formula: interface pressure = patient weight ÷ surface area supported. Sensors can also be used between the patient and the surface, but are not that reliable because of other factors such as the patient's weight, health, etc.
7. Capillary closing pressure is the pressure at which the capillaries can no longer function and if this is sustained over a period of time they burst. It is generally assumed to be 32 mmHg, but is probably more variable depending on the patient's condition.

## 3.4 AETIOLOGY

Whilst pressure and shear forces are the main causes of pressure sores, the picture is not that simple. Patients who appear to be very similar can vary in whether they develop a pressure sore or not and, while some patients will develop irreversible damage in less than 2 hours, others will not. It seems logical to conclude that other factors play a part in which patients will develop pressure sores.

Predisposing factors in the formation of pressure sores are commonly divided into two categories:

- intrinsic
- extrinsic.

### Intrinsic

This relates to internal aspects affected by the patient's physical and psychological state. Intrinsic factors affect the response mechanism and/or alter the structural components and tissue perfusion, reducing the ability of the skin and supporting tissues to respond to pressure and shear forces. Examples of intrinsic causes are listed below.

- Nutrition (see Sect. 3.5 for further information on the effect this has).
- Physical condition—may cause immobility, loss of appetite, production of sweat, loss of weight, disturbance in blood chemistry.
- Constipation—reduces nutritional intake, leads to lethargy.
- Mental state—may cause apathy, immobility, loss of appetite, loss of weight.
- Age—can affect mobility, appetite, continence, mental state, skin elasticity.
- Reduced circulation, e.g. from anaemia or peripheral vascular disease—reduces the supply of oxygen and nutrients to the tissues.
- Smoking—reduces blood flow in some patients, and reduces oxygen-carrying capacity of blood.
- Some medication—sedation immobilises patients, steroids cause thinning of the skin, cytotoxic drugs affect the immune system.
- Pain—can immobilise patients and lead to loss of appetite and fatigue.
- Diabetes—peripheral neuropathy reduces ability of patients to feel damage occurring to them, particularly in the foot region. Many diabetics suffer from circulatory problems which reduce the blood flow.
- Surgery—with particular risk to the elderly fractured femur patients (Versluysen 1986).
- Neurological deficit—particularly when it is new, such as spinal cord injury or stroke.
- The patient's sex—many surveys have found that more women than men suffer from pressure sores, but there are two schools of thought on this. The first is that, since women live longer, there are simply more women around to develop pressure damage. The second regards the difference as a result of the menopause, which can affect the skin and also makes women more susceptible to fractures that then immobilise them.

### Extrinsic

This refers to external factors, such as:

- the surface the patient is nursed on
- handling techniques
- external influences on the skin such as urine, faeces, excess talcum powder, perfume, starch from sheets, etc. affecting skin strength and Ph.

Extrinsic factors reduce the tissue tolerance by affecting the skin surface, either by weakening it, as in wet conditions, damaging it by incorrect lifting, or altering the acid balance, such as with perfumes, creams and over-frequent use of soap.

**20 MINUTES**

1. What effect do (a) extrinsic and (b) intrinsic factors have on the body?
2. Using Table 3.3, choose two patients in your caseload with pressure damage, then write down which intrinsic and extrinsic factors you consider could have contributed to pressure sore development.

| Table 3.3 | | |
|---|---|---|
| Patient | Intrinsic factors | Extrinsic factors |
| A | | |
| B | | |

**FEEDBACK**

You should have said that:

1. a. Extrinsic factors reduce tissue tolerance by weakening the skin or changing the pH balance.
   b. Intrinsic factors affect the response mechanism and tissue perfusion, reducing the ability of the skin and tissues to respond to external forces.

2. Your answer to Question 2 will depend on your patients, but check it against the lists provided in the text. You should have considered factors relating to the surface the patient is being nursed on, how the patient is moved and handled, and the patient's general condition. Were you aware of all the risk factors and how they affected the body, particularly in relation to the patient you chose, before you did this exercise?

This should have started you thinking about what causes some patients to develop pressure damage. It is probable that the more contributory factors a patient has, the more likely he is to develop a pressure sore, although this does not always happen. It is essential that any contributory factors are dealt with by the whole health care team, looking at the mental, physiological, mobility and pressure problems. Dealing with a contributory factor, in isolation, is unlikely to prevent a pressure sore, for example, providing a special mattress, but not improving the patient's physiological state if he is malnourished and anaemic. In the next two subsections, on nutrition and risk assessment tools, some of the controversies relating to predisposing factors are highlighted.

## 3.5 NUTRITION

Eating and drinking are essential to life and health. The link between nutrition and wound healing is well documented (see Reader Article 2, p. 109). Because of the effect on the body tissues of lack of nutrients, it would seem that providing nutrition is an essential tool in the attempt to prevent pressure damage occurring. Unfortunately, it is also an aspect of patient care which nursing staff in hospital have allowed to move outside their control. Elderly people require less energy intake than younger people, but for a variety of reasons their intake falls below an acceptable level (Nazarko 1993) resulting in sub-optimal nutrition.

### Effects of poor nutrition

The link between pressure sore development and poor nutrition is not universally accepted. This can be seen by the fact that it is excluded from some risk assessment tools, particularly the earlier ones.

Bergstrom & Braden (1992) draw attention to the link between protein malnutrition and pressure sore development. In direct conflict, however, other writers feel that the low protein levels in patients with pressure damage may have occurred as a result of protein leaking from the wound in the exudate (Berlowitz & Wilking 1989), in other words are caused by the sore, rather than the other way around. Many people involved in day-to-day management of high-risk patients notice that improved nutritional intake appears to help in preventing pressure damage, but more clinical research needs to be done. This is discussed in more detail later in this section. Oliver (1994; Reader Article 3) describes some of the effects that poor nutrition can have on individuals, and indeed relates them to predisposing factors in pressure sore development.

## Activity    15 MINUTES

Read Article 3 in the Reader (p. 111) and say what the two main areas are that Oliver identifies as the effects of poor nutrition, and the effects they have on a person.

. . . . . . . . . . . . . . . . . . . . . . . . . . . . . . . .

## FEEDBACK

You should have said that the two areas identified and the effects they have are:

- decline in health which can lead to physical and psychological problems which then reduce mobility
- reduced effectiveness of the immune system resulting in more infections and subsequent increase in risk of developing pressure sores.

. . . . . . . . . . . . . . . . . . . . . . . . . . . . . . . .

Nazarko (1993) quotes studies showing 7% of elderly people suffering from clinical malnutrition, those over 80 having twice the incidence of the others. She points out that this is probably the tip of the iceberg, suboptimal nutrition not being recognised in these surveys.

One element of nutrition where there is still controversy about the effects it has is vitamin C. Vitamin C is reported by McLaren (1992) to be of importance in both wound healing and pressure sore prevention, deficiency leading to reduction in wound tensile strength. She also presents some of the conflicting evidence in relation to its effect on the autoimmune system. There is also evidence of muscle weakness which leads to reduced mobility which is one of the risk factors in pressure sore formation. Vitamin C is not stored in the body, and regular daily intake is essential. Raw or lightly cooked green vegetables and fruit are good sources of vitamin C,

but as many elderly people lack these in their diet, they often have a deficiency.

Another overall effect of malnutrition is thinning of the dermis caused by the breakdown of skin collagen and again this predisposes to pressure sores by reducing skin resistance to external forces. Protein synthesis is also reduced as an effect of poor nutrition, resulting in tissue breakdown, weight loss, and reduction in subcutaneous tissue (McLaren 1992). This then makes the bony prominences more susceptible when subjected to pressure, and is one reason why these are the key areas to watch first for signs of pressure damage.

## Activity    15 MINUTES

In Reader Article 3, Oliver lists factors which contribute to poor nutrition in the community. Having read the article, list as many as you can remember.

. . . . . . . . . . . . . . . . . . . . . . . . . . . . . . . .

## FEEDBACK

You should have listed the following:

- physical condition
- money
- loneliness
- physical ability—to shop, cook or eat
- confusion
- carer support
- teeth/indigestion.

. . . . . . . . . . . . . . . . . . . . . . . . . . . . . . . .

In the acute sector, factors may be:

- pain
- nausea
- depression/feeling unwell
- inability to swallow—due to stroke or postoperatively
- dentures—loss of, not bringing them into hospital, or ill-fitting because of loss of weight
- insufficient time to eat meals
- dislike of food provided, or unsuitable, e.g. ethnic or vegetarian
- unfamiliar meal times
- inability to cut up food
- dislike of eating with company or in the day room.

Frequently the only attempt made to solve this is to provide supplementary feeds, and if these are given near a meal, they may have the opposite effect, by reducing the patient's desire for anything further to eat.

Proper nutritional assessments should be done on all patients to enable staff to identify those who are not taking in enough food, and plans of care incorporated which take into account the patients' needs and why they are not eating. An example of this is loss of or ill-fitting dentures, the latter being likely if patients have recently lost weight, which then compounds the problem. These patients should have an urgent dental referral. Some nutritional assessment tools have been developed but there needs to be a move to provide ones for specific patient groups, and for more widespread use of them.

## Activity — 30 MINUTES

Think about ways in which you could increase the likelihood of patients in your own nursing area gaining better nutrition. Make a list of at least five.

## FEEDBACK

Some strategies for dealing with problems in the hospital/nursing home sector would be as follows.

- Provide pleasant surroundings.
- Stop other medical personnel from disturbing patients at meal times—this may require reorganisation of the meal times with the kitchen, or reorganisation of ward rounds.
- Have enough staff at hand to help at meal times, and encourage relatives to come in and help if they want to.
- Involve speech therapists and dietitians where needed.
- Offer supplements at sensible times, or consider adding tasteless ones to the existing diet, particularly to soups and sweets.
- Ensure that medical staff are aware of the problems, and consider enteral or parenteral feeding.

Dextrose/saline, that favourite postoperative fare, contains calories only. It is far cheaper to feed patients, even parenterally for a short period, than it is to treat a pressure sore which has developed as a result of poor nutrition.

Community care is different but look at:

- provision of meals on wheels
- nutritional advice—perhaps by group health promotion sessions
- involvement of dentist where appropriate
- involvement of dietitian
- lunch clubs or day hospital
- supplements

- enteral feeding
- help from the family and working with social services to encourage shopping for the right food.

Overseeing nutrition in hospitals is an area which nurses threw away, and in the author's experience does not appear to be improving with the advent of streamlining and cook/chill meals. There are still areas where consultants are allowed to do ward rounds during meal times. There is often only a short time span for eating, many elderly patients are slow eaters, and nowadays trays are removed by ward orderlies who may not report whether or not patients have eaten.

Both Coates (1985) and Dickerson (1986) did surveys which found that malnutrition in patients increased in proportion to the time spent in hospital, a sobering thought if patient care is meant to be the priority. The downward spiral identified by Oliver in Reader Article 3 shows that this problem needs to be addressed, and nutrition should become a key consideration for all health professionals.

## Self-assessment — 10 MINUTES

Suggest three ways in which malnutrition may increase the risk of patients developing pressure sores.

## FEEDBACK

You should have identified the following:

- muscle weakness and reduced iron absorption leading to reduced mobility
- thinning of the dermis and reduced collagen synthesis reducing the ability of tissues to withstand pressure
- tissue breakdown and weight loss.

### 3.6 RISK ASSESSMENT

Having looked at some of the factors suspected of having a role in pressure sore formation, it is interesting to see that different assessment tools include different risk factors. A recent bulletin (Universities of Leeds & York 1995) listed the potential applications of a risk assessment tool as:

- an aid to ensure best use of limited resources, in the shape of specialised equipment

- a reminder for nurses of the risk factors when assessing patients
- to assist in correct interpretation of incidence rates in relation to number of population at risk of developing pressure sores
- as indicators of risk when trying to carry out clinical trials and compare groups of patients.

Clarke & Farrar (1992) identify 17 different tools as having been developed, possibly a measure of the fact that nurses feel that existing ones do not identify at-risk patients in their own areas. This may well be because they are expecting the tools to be predictors rather than indicators of risk. That is, they expect tools to predict who will develop a pressure sore, rather than using them in the intended way as an aide mémoire to be used in conjunction with professional judgement to highlight patients with the potential to develop pressure sores.

This section looks at four of the tools:

- Norton
- Waterlow
- Andersen
- Medley

as well as some of the problems related to using them.

## Specific tools

### Norton

The Norton assessment tool (Norton et al 1962) was the first used for risk assessment and was developed and tested on care of the elderly patients, originally to assess their general condition. Since then, many other tools have appeared, particularly for acute areas. This is because many people feel Norton is unsuitable for this group of patients because it does not include risk factors relating to acute patients. As it was devised for the elderly, this is hardly surprising, and simply represents inappropriate use when moved out of its own care setting.

It does not include nutrition, which would be important for elderly patients, but this is probably indicative of the recent importance attached to this area compared to 30 years ago. Originally anyone with a score of 14 and below was judged at risk, and there is no division into low, medium or high risk according to the score. Norton herself has since redefined the score and now anyone with a score of 16 or below is judged to be at risk. When using the tool one choice only can be made from each category. It was designed for use by nursing staff (see Table 3.4).

### Waterlow

This was devised by Waterlow in 1987 as a more comprehensive tool for assessing patients in non-geriatric wards and contains many more perceived risk factors than Norton. Waterlow herself highlights the requirements of an assessment tool as being:

- simple but accurate and comprehensive
- usable at the bedside
- usable in all hospital areas so that nurses become familiar with it
- able to fit in with the stages of planning care, namely assessment, planning, implementation and evaluation.

The tool divides patients recognised as at risk into three categories:

- low risk 10–14
- medium risk 15–19
- high risk 20 +.

When using the tool as many choices can be made from one category as necessary. For example, if a patient has oedema, clammy skin from a temperature and a discoloured area, using the skin type section of the score, he or she would score a total of 4 for this category alone. It was designed for use by nursing staff, and requires a good knowledge of individual patients to complete (see Table 3.5).

| Table 3.4 The Norton risk scale | | | | | | | | | |
|---|---|---|---|---|---|---|---|---|---|
| *Physical condition* | | *Mental state* | | *Activity* | | *Mobility* | | *Incontinence* | |
| Good | 4 | Alert | 4 | Ambulant | 4 | Full | 4 | Not/catheterised | 4 |
| Fair | 3 | Apathetic | 3 | Walks with help | 3 | Slightly limited | 3 | Occasionally | 3 |
| Poor | 2 | Confused | 2 | Chairbound | 2 | Very limited | 2 | Usually urinary | 2 |
| Very bad | 1 | Stuporous | 1 | Bedfast | 1 | Immobile | 1 | Double | 1 |
| Score: 16 or below = 'at risk' of developing pressure sores. | | | | | | | | | |

**Table 3.5** The Waterlow risk scale*

| Build/weight for height | | Skin type/visual risk area | | Sex/age | | Mobility | | Appetite | | Special risks | |
|---|---|---|---|---|---|---|---|---|---|---|---|
| Average | 0 | Healthy | 0 | Male | 1 | Fully | 0 | Average | 0 | *Tissue malnutrition, e.g.* | |
| Above average | 1 | Tissue paper | 1 | Female | 2 | Restless/fidgety | 1 | Poor | 1 | Terminal cachexia | 8 |
| Obese | 2 | Dry | 1 | 14–49 | 1 | Apathetic | 2 | Nasogastric tube/fluids only | 2 | Cardiac failure | 5 |
| Below average | 3 | Oedematous | 1 | 50–64 | 2 | Restricted | 3 | Nil by mouth/anorexic | 3 | Peripheral vascular disease | 5 |
| *Continence* | | Clammy (temp. ↑) | 1 | 65–74 | 3 | Inert/traction | 4 | | | Anaemia | 2 |
| Complete/catheterised | 0 | Discoloured | 2 | 75–80 | 4 | Chairbound | 5 | | | Smoking | 1 |
| Occasional incontinence | 1 | Broken spot | 3 | 81+ | 5 | | | | | *Neurological deficit, e.g.* | |
| Catheterised/incontinence of faeces | 2 | | | | | | | | | Diabetes, MS, CVA, motor/sensory paraplegia | 4–6 |
| Doubly incontinent | 3 | | | | | | | | | *Major surgery/trauma* | |
| | | | | | | | | | | Orthopaedic—below waist, spinal | 5 |
| | | | | | | | | | | On table > 2 hours | 5 |
| | | | | | | | | | | *Medication* | |
| | | | | | | | | | | Cytotoxics, high-dose steroids, anti-inflammatory | 4 |

* Ring scores in table. Several scores per category can be used.
Score: 10+ = at risk; 15+ = high risk; 20+ = very high risk.

## Andersen

This was developed in Denmark by Andersen et al (1982) for patients being admitted to hospital with acute conditions, and was for non-medical personnel, so that quick assessments could be made and preventive strategies implemented. More than one choice can be made from each category, but there is no division into degrees of risk. Any single one factor on the absolute column puts the patient at risk (see Table 3.6).

| Risk criteria | |
|---|---|
| Absolute (score 2) | Relative (score 1) |
| Unconsciousness | Age (> 70 years) |
| Dehydration | Restricted mobility |
| Paralysis | Incontinence |
| | Pronounced emaciation |
| | Redness over bony prominences |

**Table 3.6** The Andersen risk scale

## Medley

This tool, again, was devised with more categories for patients by Williams in 1991. More than one choice can be made for each category and where scores jump from 4 to 6, for example in the activity and mobility range, the nurse can award 5 if she feels there is an overlap of factors. It splits at-risk patients into three groups:

- low risk 0–9
- medium risk 10–19
- high risk 20–36.

It requires a knowledge of the patient, and is designed for nursing staff (see Table 3.7).

## Comparison of risk assessment tools

A quick look at the four tools considered above will show two basic differences. These are:

- the varying number of risk factors considered
- the fact that with three of them, the higher the score the higher the risk, while with Norton, the lower the score the higher the risk.

**Table 3.7** The Medley risk scale

| | Score | | Score |
|---|---|---|---|
| **Activity—ambulation** | | **Nutritional status** | |
| Ambulant without assistance | 0 | Good (eats/drinks/or nasogastric feeds) | 0 |
| Ambulant with assistance | 2 | Fair (insufficient intake to maintain weight) | 1 |
| Chairfast (longer than 12 hours) | 4 | Poor (eats/drinks very little) | 2 |
| Bedfast (longer than 12 hours) | 6 | Very poor (unable or refuses to eat; emaciated) | 3 |
| **Skin condition** | | **Incontinence—bladder** | |
| Healthy (clear and moist) | 0 | None or catheterised | 0 |
| Rashes or abrasions | 2 | Occasional (less than two per 24 hours) | 1 |
| Decreased turgor; dry skin, advanced age | 4 | Usually (more than two per 24 hours) | 2 |
| Oedema and/or redness | 6 | Total (no control) | 3 |
| Pressure sore involved | | | |
| **Predisposing disease** | | **Incontinence—bowel** | |
| No involvement | 0 | None | 0 |
| Chronic stable | 1 | Occasional (formed stool) | 1 |
| Acute or chronic unstable | 2 | Usually (with formed stool) | 2 |
| Terminal or grave | 3 | Total (no control) | 3 |
| **Mobility—range of motion** | | **Pain** | |
| Full active range of motion | 0 | None | 0 |
| Moves with limited assistance | 2 | Mild | 1 |
| Moves only with assistance | 4 | Intermittent | 2 |
| Immobile | 6 | Severe | 3 |
| **Level of consciousness (to commands)** | | | |
| Alert | 0 | **Patient risk score:** | |
| Lethargic/confusion | 1 | 0–9 = low risk | |
| Semi-comatose (absence of response to stimuli) | 2 | 10–19 = medium risk | |
| Comatose (absence of response to stimuli) | 3 | 20–36 = high risk | |

Staff transferring patients from one care setting to another need to know which tool a risk assessment refers to. For example, score of 17 would indicate the following:

- Norton, no risk
- Waterlow, medium risk
- Medley, medium risk
- Andersen, at risk.

**Activity**     **45 MINUTES**

Using the four tools and Table 3.8, tick off in each of the columns which tools contain which risk factors, Once completed look carefully and state how many factors are recognised by all four tools.

**FEEDBACK**

You should have noted that the only two factors identified by all four tools are mobility and continence. Given the importance attached to shear forces and their role in pressure sore development, it is interesting to note the total exclusion of this category from all tools. A section on lifting would cover this. However, the wide disparity of factors would suggest that far more needs to be known about absolute risk factors before any more tools are added to the extending list.

## Which factors are relevant?

Bridel (1994) looks at a series of questions relating to risk assessment tools. Among them are the following.

1. How has the choice been made to include certain factors in the tools?
2. Are these factors recognised as key prognostic factors for developing pressure sores?
3. How successful are these calculators at predicting who is at risk?

These are key questions, and will be looked at one by one.

### *How has the choice been made to include certain factors in the tools?*

Bridel (1994) looked at several different tools, and how the authors had chosen whether or not to include certain factors in them. She found that factors were selected by a variety of methods, not all of them very scientific. Examples of how selection was made include:

- after discussion on research among staff
- on the basis of clinical experience
- after a literature review
- after discussion with medical colleagues.
- developed for use in specific areas with a view to researching its effectiveness.

Strictly speaking, this last is the only response which would validate a choice, as it suggests that factors have been selected, and research will then be done into their effectiveness in recognising patients at risk.

| Table 3.8 | Norton | Waterlow | Andersen | Medley |
|---|---|---|---|---|
| Mobility | | | | |
| Nutrition | | | | |
| Age | | | | |
| Sex | | | | |
| Activity | | | | |
| Special risks | | | | |
| Medication | | | | |
| Skin type | | | | |
| Weight | | | | |
| Continence | | | | |
| Physical condition | | | | |
| Mental condition | | | | |
| Shear forces | | | | |
| Consciousness | | | | |
| Pain | | | | |

### *Are these factors recognised as key prognostic factors for developing pressure sores?*

How to choose the factors which should be included in risk assessment tools is dependent on this second question raised by Bridel.

This is of course where problems arise. It is not so many years since bad nursing care and pressure were the only two accepted causes of pressure sores, as has already been looked at. That other factors contribute is now recognised, but lack of agreement on how important these factors are has been shown by the previous activity. The Andersen score contains very few categories and is a very simple scoring system, yet a study of 3571 patients identified 600 patients at risk using the score, and 2916 not at risk (Andersen et al 1982). Of these groups, 40 patients identified as at risk went on to develop pressure sores, and the higher the risk score (2 being the minimum required to be at risk and 11 the maximum which could be scored) the more likely a patient was to be in the group that developed sores. Full details of preventive action taken are not discussed, and obviously this would affect results, but it was noted that the overall incidence of pressure sores was 20% for those on normal mattresses, and 6% for those on pressure-relieving systems.

Of the 2916 identified as not being at risk, only 5 developed pressure sores. As one of the criticisms levelled at assessment tools is that they over-predict, it is interesting to note that many patients in this study were not at risk, and of the 5 who developed sores, 2 had not been re-assessed following acute episodes, and 3 had been incorrectly assessed. This raises the question of how relevant it is to include all the factors which some of the other tools include, especially as the more complex the tool, the longer it takes the nurse to assess the patient. There needs to be more effort put into trying to look statistically at the effect each factor has on development of pressure sores, so that the key ones can be identified and used as the prime indicators. A problem with this of course is that, ethically, trials cannot be conducted where pressure relief is denied to at-risk patients, so it may prove difficult to pinpoint causes.

### *How successful are these calculators at predicting who is at risk?*

Bridel's third question relating to success of predicting who is at risk ties in with the above. The validity of a tool is dependent on its specificity and sensitivity; ideally there should be no under- or over-prediction. No tool achieves this, but more work needs to be done to identify which tools perform best.

### Judging a tool's performance

Two main indicators exist in relation to looking at the ability of a tool to do the job it is supposed to do. They are:

- reliability—the degree of consistency with which a tool measures the attribute it is supposed to be measuring
- validity—the 'degree to which a tool measures what it is supposed to measure' (Towey & Erland 1988).

Two further indicators make up the validity factor. These are:

- specificity—the ability of the tool to predict those who will develop a condition
- sensitivity—the correct prediction of those who will not develop a condition.

Unless a tool can be found to have a high level of accuracy in these areas, there can be little value in using it to try to find out who is likely to develop a pressure sore, or as a means of allocating resources. However, other factors can affect these measurements. Treece & Treece (1982) state the possible causes of tools failing to achieve reliability and validity as:

- an error or deficiency in the tool itself
- inconsistency among those using the tool.

Sensitivity and specificity assume that tools are predictors, but initially their role was as indicators, to alert staff to the potential for a problem. Is this why there are now problems with their use, do we expect too much of them? What has happened to clinical judgement and experience, which are valuable tools in their own right? The bulletin by the Universities of Leeds and York (1995) concludes that 'there is little evidence that using a pressure sore risk scale is better than clinical judgement or that it improves outcomes', a sobering thought when one looks at all the tools that exist, and the time spent by nurses on assessment. Does this also suggest that nurses who have not yet developed clinical judgement are the ones being asked to assess the patients? However, it is likely that assessment tools do meet one of the criteria mentioned at the beginning of this section, and that is that they remind nurses during assessment of the risk factors.

### Activity                                              2 HOURS

This activity is to help you look at some of the issues highlighted above. Take each of the case histories given in Box 3.1 and score the patients using each of the four scoring systems shown in this section, then ask a friend to do the same. Compare the categories of risk into which each tool places the patients. Were

**Box 3.1** Case histories

**1. Mrs A**

Mrs A, who is 74 years old, was admitted with a fractured femur, and is now 3 days postoperative. She is withdrawn, taking small amounts of diet and fluid, immobilised and on bed rest, catheterised and constipated. She has a temperature from a chest infection for which she is having antibiotics. Her haemoglobin was 9.2 g/dl preoperatively, but 11.4 g/dl postoperatively following blood transfusion. She takes steroids which control her arthritis, and is overweight. She has thin, papery skin and discoloured heels. She has postoperative pain when moved.

**2. Mr B**

Mr B is 31 years old and has been paraplegic since the age of 20. He is catheterised and has a microlax enema on alternate days. He has appropriate pressure-relieving equipment for his needs in his wheelchair and on his bed. Normally he eats very well and does wheelchair sports. He lives with his girlfriend, but is largely self-caring, and transfers himself from wheelchair to bed. He has a haemoglobin level of 14.2 g/dl. The district nurse visits for bladder washouts because of problems with his catheter blocking, and providing these are done regularly he has no problems.

there differences in the scores of you and your colleague? Did you have problems with any of the categories? With the exception of Norton, you can use more than one factor from each category.

● ● ● ● ● ● ● ● ● ● ● ● ● ● ● ● ● ● ● ● ● ● ● ● ● ● ● ● ● ● ● ● ● ● ● ●

# FEEDBACK

## Case history 1

Norton score:

| | |
|---|---|
| Physical condition | 2 (poor) |
| Mental state | 3 (apathetic) |
| Activity | 1 (bedfast) |
| Mobility | 1 (immobile) |
| Incontinence | 4 (none) |

Total 11 = at risk.

Waterlow score:

| | |
|---|---|
| Build | 2 (obese) |
| Continence | 0 |
| Skin | 1 (tissue paper), 2 (discoloured) |
| Mobility | 2 (apathetic), 4 (traction) |
| Sex/age | 2 (female), 3 (74 years) |
| Appetite | 1 (poor) |
| Special risks | 5 (major trauma), 4 (steroids) |

Total 26 = very high risk.

Andersen score:

| | |
|---|---|
| Age | 1 (> 70 years) |
| Mobility | 1 (restricted) |
| Redness | 1 |

Total 3 = at risk.

Medley score:

| | |
|---|---|
| Activity | 6 (bedfast) |
| Skin | 4 (dry skin and age), 6 (pressure sore—heel) |
| Predisposing disease | 1 (arthritis—chronic) |
| Mobility | 6 (immobile) |
| Consciousness | 1 (lethargic) |
| Nutrition | 2 (poor) |
| Incontinence—bladder | 0 (catheter) |
| Incontinence—bowels | 0 (at the moment) |
| Pain | 2 (intermittent) |

Total 28 = high risk.

All tools recognised this patient as being at risk, but clinical judgement would have told a nurse the same. Did you notice the time it took to use the different tools which, whilst differing in their estimation of degree of risk, all came to the same conclusion regarding this patient?

## Case history 2

Norton score:

| | |
|---|---|
| Physical condition | 4 (good) or 3 (fair)* |
| Mental state | 4 (alert) |
| Activity | 2 (chairbound) |
| Mobility | 3 (slightly immobile) or 2 (very limited)* |
| Incontinence | 4 (none) |

Total 15–17 depending on scores marked with an asterisk = risk or no risk.

Waterlow score:

| | |
|---|---|
| Build | 0 (average) |
| Continence | 0 (catheter) |
| Skin | 0 (healthy) |
| Mobility | 3 (restricted) and/or 5 (chairbound)* |
| Sex/age | 1 (male), 1 (< 49 years) |
| Appetite | 0 |
| Special risks | 4–6 (paraplegic)* |

Total 11–16 depending on score marked with an asterisk = risk or high risk.

Andersen score:

| | |
|---|---|
| Paralysis | 2 |
| Mobility | 1* (restricted) |

Total 2–3 depending on whether score marked with an asterisk is included = at risk.

Medley score:

| | |
|---|---|
| Activity | 4 (chair) |
| Skin | 0 (healthy) |
| Predisposing disease | 0 (none) |
| Mobility | 2 (immobile) |
| Consciousness | 2 (limited assistance) |
| Nutrition | 0 (good) |
| Incontinence—bladder | 0 (catheter) |
| Incontinence—bowels | 0 |
| Pain | 0 |

Total 6 = low risk.

This assessment may have caused you more problems and disagreement with your colleague. The variations in the risk factors are more noticeable, and can it really be said that this patient is in fact at risk in his present alert and healthy state, with all the correct equipment? Disagreement on the degree of mobility, i.e. whether you consider him as very restricted or quite mobile, may well be affected by where you work. Again, notice the difference in time that each assessment tool took to use.

● ● ● ● ● ● ● ● ● ● ● ● ● ● ● ● ● ● ● ● ● ● ● ● ● ● ● ● ● ● ● ● ● ● ●

The overall findings from the Universities of Leeds & York (1995) in relation to using risk assessment tools are:

- Many have been developed using possible risk factors, not proven ones.
- They should not be moved out of specific care settings if devised for those areas.
- No published evaluation of the use of tools in reducing pressure sore incidence exists.
- Great variations are achieved in results using the same tools, depending on the assessment methods and the care setting.

## When to assess?

Despite these findings in the 1995 report, patients do need assessing for risk so that interventions can be made. Whether these assessments are by experienced clinical judgement or use of assessment tools, the latter do at least provide a structured framework in which to carry out and record the results of the procedure.

Although knowledge about key factors and the critical time in which pressure sores develop is still open to discussion, baselines need to be set, and one such is the 2-hour margin commonly taken as the time span in which pressure damage can occur. As has already been discussed, amount and time of pressure loading remain open to debate. Using this it would be wise to set a standard that patients at least have a preliminary assessment within 2 hours of admission to any health care setting, although this is not feasible in the community where staff have to rely on discharge information from hospital staff, cannot always visit within this time scale, or indeed do not always know that patients have been discharged until 24–48 hours after they have arrived home.

A tool such as Andersen can be useful, as it is quick to use, as was shown in the last activity, and therefore ideal for busy areas such as accident and emergency departments. If assessment can be done before this, for example by ambulance personnel, this is even better (McClemont et al 1991). In these cases, areas to which the patient is being transferred can be alerted before the patient arrives, which enables staff to have a preventive plan in action and acquire any equipment they may need. The operating staff should always be alerted to patients in the risk category so that they also may make the most effective use of their often limited resources and, where possible, make provision for patients undergoing some of the longer procedures. It should be remembered that a few patients assessed as not at risk may in fact be at risk, e.g. during a period of surgery, typically maxillofacial operations, which can take many hours. During this time, the patient is unmoving on a hard surface, and often has a lowered blood pressure as a result of the anaesthetic, reducing the blood flow to the peripheries.

Community patients should be assessed during the first visit by the district nurse, and thereafter when their condition or home circumstances change. Some areas also reassess on a weekly basis, which may pick up more subtle changes and alter a patient's risk category up or down. The major changes which should highlight the necessity to reassess patients are:

- surgery
- deterioration in general condition, mental or physical
- loss of appetite
- presence of infection (wound, chest and urinary are common ones)
- change in care setting; transfer to community might mean lower nursing input
- cardiac arrest or collapse from other causes.

Failure to carry out a reassessment can result in patients developing pressure sores because their increased susceptibility has gone unnoticed.

## Self-assessment                    3 HOURS

1. Take 10 minutes to note down how and when you think risk assessment tools should be used.

2. Take the next six patients you see in your caseload, allocate to each of them an identity

number to ensure confidentiality and when you have time check through their nursing notes and answer the following questions for each patient.

a. Was the patient assessed within 2 hours of admission or, in the case of patients in the community, on the first visit?
b. Has the patient been assessed within the last week?
c. If the patient has had a major change in the last week, such as surgery or start of a chest infection, was he or she reassessed then?

Note: you should clear this activity with your manager, as it comprises a small audit involving patients.

## FEEDBACK

Risk assessment tools should be used as indicators of risk in conjunction with professional and clinical knowledge. They should be used to plan preventive strategies, and alert other care areas to the need to provide equipment for the patient on transfer. They should be used within 2 hours of admission to hospital or care home, or on first community visit, or when there are any major changes in care setting or condition.

The exercise with your own patients may have highlighted shortfalls in your assessment procedure. It may also have highlighted problems with your nursing records; for example, were you able to retrieve the information easily? If you have a policy or standards stating that assessment occurs within 2 hours of admission, or on the first visit, you should be able to audit that against the nursing record. Any shortfalls identified should be discussed with the rest of your team.

## Education

Already identified as a factor affecting a tool's usefulness, is the consistency with which people use it. One of the previous activities may also have highlighted this as a problem. A key to overcoming this is education, not only on why and when to use the tools, but also on how. This is often not done. There have been surveys showing some variations achieved by staff using assessment tools (Bridel 1993), which has obvious implications for the reliability and validity of the tools. Additionally, as has been seen, some tools allow only one factor to be selected from each section, while others allow as many as necessary.

Nurses should be educated in the use and interpretation of tools within their own area, so that everyone has the same comprehension of how to apply the categories, particularly loss of mobility, general health, etc. Doing this may in fact open up the whole arena of risk assessment for discussion in that care setting, and increase awareness of both the problems and importance of this action for both patients and staff. As well as education into the use of tools, all aspects of pressure sore prevention must also be covered, but it is use of the tools which is often neglected.

Some options on effective education will be looked at in the section on prevention including education of patient and/or carer (p. 57). In cases where concerns are raised over pressure sore development, it is now expected that nurses will have assessed a patient, acted on that assessment, and recorded this information in the care plan. It is therefore advisable to use a tool which is as reliable and valid as possible for that care setting. Local policies should be in place for time scales relating to assessment and action taken depending on the score. However, it should be remembered that more than the tool should be used to determine patient care.

### Self-assessment    20 MINUTES

1. Give a definition of validity.
2. Give a definition of reliability.
3. Which two factors were the only ones recognised by all four assessment tools used in this text?
4. Which two factors did Treece & Treece (1982) identify as factors which caused tools to fail to achieve reliability and validity?

## FEEDBACK

You should have said the following.

1. Reliability is the degree of consistency with which a tool measures the attribute it is supposed to measure.
2. Validity is the degree to which a tool measures what it is supposed to measure.
3. The only two consistent factors in each tool were continence and mobility.
4. The two factors identified by Treece & Treece as reasons for tools failing were, an error or deficiency in the tool itself, and inconsistency among those using the tool.

## SUMMARY

This section should have given you the following knowledge:

- skin and its vascular system are where pressure damage has the greatest effect

- duration and type of pressure damage have an impact on whether or not pressure sores develop

- intrinsic and extrinsic factors combined contribute to pressure sore development

- risk assessment tools should be used to assist in allocation of resources, correct interpretation of incidence data and as a reminder to nurses of risk factors when assessing patients.

### REFERENCES

Andersen K E, Jensen O, Kvorning S A, Bach E 1982 Prevention of pressure sores by identifying patients at risk. British Medical Journal 284: 1370–1372

Bader D 1990 Pressure sores clinical practice and scientific approach. Macmillan, London

Barton A, Barton M 1981 The management and prevention of pressure sores. Faber & Faber, London

Benbow M 1992 Keeping the pressure off. Nursing the Elderly (May–June): 17–19

Bergstrom N, Braden B J 1992 A prospective study of pressure sore risk among the institutionalised elderly. Journal of American Geriatric Society 40(8): 747–758

Bergstrom N, Braden B J, Laguzza A, Holman V 1987 The Braden scale for predicting pressure sores. Nursing Research 36(4): 206–210

Berlowitz D, Wilking S 1989 Risk factors for pressure sores; a comparison of cross sectional and cohort data. Journal of American Geriatric Society 37(11): 1043–1050

Bridel J 1993 The aetiology of pressure sores. Journal of Wound Care 2(4): 230–238

Bridel J 1994 Risk assessment. Journal of Tissue Viability 4(3): 84–85

Burman P M S, O'Dea K 1994 Measuring pressure. Journal of Wound Care 3(2): 83–86

Clarke M, Farrar S 1992 Comparison of risk calculators. In: Harding K G, Leaper D L, Turner T D (eds) Proceedings of the First European Conference in Advanced Wound Management. Macmillan, London

Coates V 1985 Are they being served? Royal College of Nursing, London

Collier M 1994 The skin. Wound Care Society Education Leaflet No 2. Wound Care Society, Northampton

Davies K 1994 Prevention of pressure sores. British Journal of Nursing 3(21): 1099–1104

Dickerson J 1986 Hospital induced malnutrition—a cause for concern. Professional Nurse (August): 293–296

Kosiak M 1959 Aetiology and pathology of ischaemic ulcers. Archives of Physical Medicine and Rehabilitation 40: 62–69

Krouskop M 1983 A synthesis of the factors which contribute to pressure sore formation. Medical Hypothesis 11: 255–267

Landis E 1930 Studies of capillary blood pressure in human skin. Heart 15: 209

McClemont E, Woodcock N, Oliver S, Hinton C, Preston K, Phillips J 1991 The Lincoln experience, part one. Journal of Tissue Viability 2(4): 114–117

McLaren S 1992 Nutrition and wound healing. Journal of Wound Care 1(3): 45–55

Nazarko L 1993 Nutritional problems in nursing homes. Nursing Standard 7(27): 33–35

Norton D 1989 Calculating the risk, reflections on the Norton score. Decubitus (August): 24–31

Norton D, McLaren R, Exton-Smith A N 1962 An investigation of geriatric nursing problems in hospital. National Corporation for the Care of Old People, London

Towey A, Erland S 1988 Validity and reliability of an assessment tool for pressure ulcer risk. Decubitus 1(2): 40–48

Treece E, Treece J 1982 Elements of research in nursing, 3rd edn. C V Mosby, Missouri

Universities of Leeds & York 1995 Effective health care. Churchill Livingstone, Edinburgh, vol 2, no 1

Versluysen M 1986 How elderly patients with femur factures develop pressure sores in hospital. British Medical Journal 292(17 May): 1311–1313

Waterlow J 1987 Calculating the risk. Nursing Times 83(39): 58–60

Williams C 1991 Comparing Norton and Medley. Nursing Times 87(36): 66–68

# 4 Prevention of pressure sores

Having discussed the causes of pressure sores, and how to identify patients at risk of developing them, it is essential to recognise the different strategies which can be used in their prevention, in addition to improving mental and physiological status. This is a key area, and there is no doubt that it is preferable to prevent pressure sores rather than to allow them to occur, particularly from the patient's point of view. Cohesive multidisciplinary strategies, encompassing the whole episode of a patient's care, are the foundations for effective pressure sore prevention.

## LEARNING OUTCOMES

At the end of this section you will be able to identify:

- the different types of equipment available to provide pressure relief
- the role of the clinical nurse specialist in pressure sore prevention
- the importance of education in a prevention programme
- the importance of communication in discharge planning
- aspects to include in a prevention policy.

Davies (1994) gives an overview of pressure sore prevention and identifies the key skills needed by staff as:

- a knowledge of the aetiology of pressure sores
- an awareness of the factors that increase the risk of developing pressure sores
- the ability to assess who is at risk of developing pressure sores
- anticipation of problems which may occur
- the knowledge to prevent pressure sores occurring
- the ability to apply knowledge to clinical practice.

Some of these have already been covered in Section 3; the remainder will be looked at in this section.

## 4.1 CHOOSING THE RIGHT EQUIPMENT

This is a minefield as there are many different systems on the market. Young (1992) stresses the importance of checking that the equipment has been evaluated

for its effectiveness before marketing. It is also important that staff do not feel that providing equipment will solve all their problems. It is essential that education is combined with the provision of equipment. There are numerous types of equipment on the market, with more arriving each week, and as the main users, nursing staff need to know:

- how pressure-relieving systems work including quick deflation for resuscitation
- how to match patients and equipment
- the most cost-effective ways of obtaining equipment
- who to contact for repair and maintenance.

### How systems work

In Section 3, the effect and types of pressure were discussed, and it may be useful to review this at this stage, before looking at ways in which equipment can reduce the effects of pressure.

---

**Self-assessment**      5 MINUTES

Complete the following sentences.

1. Pressure causes _____ of the vascular system which results in _____ of the capillaries and consequent damage to the _____ .

2. Shear _____ the tissues, and damages the _____ matrix thus removing one of the main _____ mechanisms for protecting the tissues.

. . . . . . . . . . . . . . . . . . . . . . . . . . . . . . . . . . . . .

### FEEDBACK

You should have answered with the following words or their equivalent.

1. Pressure causes occlusion of the vascular system which results in bursting of the capillaries and consequent damage to the tissues.
2. Shear disrupts the tissues and damages the collagen/elastin matrix thus removing one of the main defence mechanisms for protecting the tissues.

The important thing to remember is that it is the combination of pressure and distortion which causes the most serious damage in physiologically compromised patients.

● ● ● ● ● ● ● ● ● ● ● ● ● ● ● ● ● ● ● ● ● ● ● ● ● ● ● ● ● ● ●

## How pressure relief is obtained

The principle behind any pressure-relief strategy is spreading the load and/or relieving the pressure at regular intervals (Dealey 1995). At-risk patients left to sit in chairs can develop deeper more serious sores than those nursed in bed because a greater pressure is being exerted on a smaller surface area, the buttocks. A patient lying in bed has the pressure distributed over a greater surface area, but this is also why the bony prominences are the danger points, as they take a greater share of the load than the rest of the body. This is another reason why it is important to assess patients for risk of pressure sore development. Some risk assessment tools make recommendations as to the type of equipment you should use for patients in different categories, but these are often too simplistic. Additionally, it is essential that all patients on equipment are reassessed regularly at least once a week as their requirements may have changed up or down. Dealey (1995; Reader Article 4) recommends daily assessment, but this is not always realistic and would not be possible in the community. Flow charts can be a useful aid to selecting equipment and can be geared to specific areas and what is available. An example is given in Reader Article 4 (p. 117).

## Pressure-relieving equipment

Pressure-relieving equipment falls into two main groups:

- pressure reducing
- pressure relieving.

There are also two types of support: mattress overlays and mattress replacements. Overlays are designed to go on top of ordinary mattresses, while mattress replacements completely replace the ordinary mattress. There are also a few highly sophisticated systems in which the mattress is incorporated into a special bed frame.

### Pressure-reducing surfaces

These increase the area of the body in contact with the surface, thereby spreading the load and reducing the effects of pressure. See Reader Article 4 (p. 116) for an illustration of this effect. All systems have recommended maximum weights and information about these can be obtained from the companies marketing them.

**Fibre-filled overlays** (Plate 5, between pp. 22 and 23.) These have a limited life span, especially if sent to the laundry too often. Some can mould to the patient's body to such an extent that the filling is displaced resulting in very little effect on pressure. This is more common in care settings where they are left in situ for a long time. They are suitable for low-risk patients.

**Foam overlays.** These usually consist of slashed or cubed foam, which is said to reduce the effects of pressure further by allowing for movement. They are not suitable for heavy patients.

**Foam mattresses** (Plate 6, between pp. 22 and 23.) There are many different types, with varying foam densities, some with a combination of different foams, some with slashed or squared foam, some with foam inserts. They are also available in different depths. Varying levels of support are provided, depending on the mattress.

All of the above should be covered in vapour-permeable, multistretch covers, which can be washed in soap and water. This ensures reduction in risks of cross-infection, increased life-expectancy for the product, and continuation of pressure relief, even though there is a cover on the equipment. Plastic covers, once often used in hospitals, can still be seen in some areas, but have no give in them, producing a hammocking effect. Hammocking occurs when the cover has no elastic properties and forms a hammock shape which then prevents the patient contacting and benefiting from the underlying protective mattress.

**Gel support systems.** These contain a polymer gel which is viscous, and some have a combination of gel and foam. They are often used in theatre as there is no problem with taking X-rays through them, and they are not too bulky. They are, however, heavy. They have washable outer covers.

All patients on any of the above systems will still need regular repositioning to relieve the pressure; this can be turning or the more appropriate 30° tilt. This is a system, again based on spreading pressure over a larger surface area, which requires six or seven pillows. It is usually extremely comfortable for the patient, if correctly done, and patients can be left for longer periods than when simply turned because high pressures are not applied to the pressure points, such as the hip bones. This method is also effective when no special pressure-relieving system is in use and is a cheaper option. See Reader Article 5 (p. 118) for an explanatory leaflet on doing this. The critical points to consider to check the effectiveness of the position are that you can slide your hand under the patient as far as the sacrum, and both heels should be completely free of pressure.

**Water support systems.** Water can be found in overlays or mattresses, but is a heavy medium and there is a risk of punctures. Water-filled supports have given way in most areas to some of the new pressure-relieving mattress systems. Water is not effective as a pressure-reducing system unless it covers a large area, where the principle is that it equalises the pressures applied to the tissues. Water-filled gloves for heels do not meet this criterion.

**Air-filled mattresses.** Pressure-reducing mattresses are filled with static air which is pumped in and then adjusted to the weight of the individual patient. They need regular checks to ensure that no air has been lost, they can puncture, and education is needed on how to adjust them, which is critical. They are as good as the person using them.

**Low air loss supports.** These are overlays or mattresses electrically operated to fill them with air which is constantly replaced and escapes through small holes in the mattress. They should be adjusted for individual patients, and some systems can be more finely adjusted to different parts of the body. At the upper end of this scale there are complete beds incorporating the mattresses (Plate 7, between pp. 22 and 23), in which the whole position of the patient can be adjusted. Level of support is very variable, depending on the system chosen. Mattresses can cater for heavier patients than overlays.

**Air-fluidised supports.** These use the most sophisticated system, consisting of silicone-covered glass beads through which air is pumped to keep them constantly moving, giving a fluid effect. They come as a complete specialised bed. Excess moisture is absorbed by the bed and filtered to the bottom in clumps of beads where it can be removed. The bed can be switched off to give a static surface for carrying out nursing procedures on the patient. These beds are extremely heavy, and require comprehensive maintenance. If going into a private house or an upstairs ward it is essential that the floor is capable of sustaining the weight. The overall pressure to which the patient is subjected is about 11 mmHg. This bed also has several features which benefit patients with wounds, by reducing the stress and modifying the catabolic response (Ryan 1990).

Patients on all these systems need to be checked for pressure damage, but some will not need turning.

## Pressure-relieving systems

In these the equipment moves under the patient, thus reducing the amount of pressure being applied to any one point at regular intervals (see Reader Article 4, p. 116, for an illustration of this).

**Alternating systems.** These are overlays and mattresses where air is pumped by motor, and the same air is then circulated around the system, causing the cells which lie lengthways across the mattress to inflate and deflate under the patient. Overlays go on top of the bed mattress, and mattresses go directly onto the bed base. Different cell cycles exist in terms of cycle time and numbers of cells inflated/deflated. For example, alternate cells may be inflated/deflated, or one cell in three. Some of the mattresses are more sophisticated than others and have an extra layer of base cells to prevent bottoming out by the patient, and some have sensors which adjust to the patient's weight if the patient moves on the bed. Bottoming out is the process by which patients sink too far into the bed and end up resting on the underlying surface. Many of these systems can be turned off but remain inflated and static for a period so that patients can be transferred to another department or ward. If this facility did not exist and the mattresses deflated, the patient would end up lying on the bed base. Plate 8 (between pp. 22 and 23) shows an example of a mattress replacement.

**Airwave system.** This is a type of alternating system where three cells work on a regular cycle of one inflated, one deflated and one in between. The three cells at the head of the bed do not deflate. Very high and very low pressures are achieved throughout the cycle. Wound healing is said to be enhanced on this system, and in fact the case history considered in Section 7 appears to support this. Patients on these systems should be checked for signs of pressure damage, but require greatly reduced turning schedules.

Article 4 in the Reader (p. 116) lists some of the systems which come into the categories considered above, but by no means all, showing what a minefield selecting the correct equipment could be. Before using any system you need to know the maximum weight it can take, whether it is an overlay or mattress replacement, and what sort of patient it is designed for, low or high risk, or with pressure sores already.

## Activity                                    30 MINUTES

Using the lists and information in Reader Article 4, and those given in the text, select one of your own patients who is on a pressure-relieving/reducing mattress, then answer the following questions.

1. Is it an overlay or a mattress?

2. What type of system is it, pressure reducing or pressure relieving?

3. Did you consider either of the following when choosing the equipment:
   a. patient's weight
   b. patient's risk score
   c. any existing pressure damage.

4. Do you still consider this the most suitable equipment for this patient?

## FEEDBACK

Your answers will vary depending on the patient chosen. They may have shown an increase in your knowledge after reading this section. You may find that equipment choice is based on what is available rather than patient need, and the patient may be on equipment which is too sophisticated or too simple, both of which represent improper use of resources. Perhaps you feel that a flow chart may help to rationalise equipment choice for patients in your area.

## Seating

Patients are often provided with mattresses or overlays and then allowed to sit unprotected on chairs, yet as has been explained at the beginning of this section sitting exerts a higher pressure than lying down, and is therefore very hazardous for at-risk patients. Cushions are available and come in the following categories.

- Pressure reducing—fibre, gel, gel and foam and air. There are also some highly specialised ones available through the wheelchair services for patients assessed as having special needs. Plate 9 (between pp. 22 and 23) shows an example of a foam pressure-reducing cushion.
- Pressure-relieving alternating cushions are also on the market, but have problems of electrical supply, or bulky batteries.

Some of the most effective systems for sitting patients out are the static air-filled products, providing they are correctly adjusted, but some patients, for example ones who have had bilateral amputation, may find them unstable. Cushions chosen for wheelchairs do not always perform well if transferred to armchairs, as the dimensions, sitting position of the patient and underlying surface can all affect the cushion's performance. There are armchairs being made now which have pressure-reducing cushions built into them. If in doubt, it is best to consult your local expert who may be an occupational therapist or physiotherapist with specialist seating knowledge.

## Other options

It is important not to lose sight of simple practices and methods for reducing pressure amid all this technology. Simple measures combined with regular turning and moving patients include:

- Bed cradles to relieve the pressure on heels from the weight of the bedclothes.

- Ensuring that the sheets are not tucked in too tightly, which also increases heel pressures.
- Ensuring that any basic mattresses are not sagging or bottomed out and meet the DoH requirements of being at least 5 inches thick. Mattresses, including those in the community, should be turned on a regular weekly basis; overlays should be turned from head to foot if they do not have two operational sides. Some companies now label their mattresses with numbers so that, for example, in week 1 the number 1 should be at the head of the bed and in week 2 number 2, and so on, enabling staff to keep a check on the system.
- Not using drawsheets or plastic sheets, as the more there is between the patient and the pressure-relieving surface, the less effective it is likely to be.
- Not using plastic chairs without some protection for the patient.
- Having a mattress replacement programme within the life span of the chosen mattresses.
- Use of the 30° tilt (Reader 5).

## Choosing equipment

The first consideration is patient criteria. Article 4 in the Reader (p. 116) discusses factors relating to selection of equipment for patients in the hospital sector. Additional factors in the community might be:

- patient has a double bed and still sleeps with spouse
- input by carer
- nursing service or home care input
- patient compliance
- pets, who may damage the systems by puncturing them.

Other criteria include:

- budget available
- clinical data relating to performance of equipment
- expected life span of mattress
- maintenance and costs.

Clinical trials are quoted as the yardstick for measuring effectiveness of products, but O'Dea (1994) points out the many pitfalls in relation to this when looking at pressure relieving equipment, not least the nature of the question being asked (see Box 4.1), bearing in mind that these systems are also used for healing pressure sores. Additionally there would be ethical problems in relation to placing some at-risk patients on pressure-relieving products and not others. Once launched, products often go through a period of adjustment in relation to user comments, unlike drugs. For this reason it is important to have a way of evaluating equipment for your own area

> **Box 4.1** What is the question?
>
> - Wound healing rates?
> - Effects on sleep?
> - Role in pain relief?
> - Effects on tissue perfusion?
> - Effects on fluid balance?
> - Effects on metabolism?
> - Thermoregulation?
> - Special needs for children?
> - Air-fluidised therapy for neonates?
> - Prevention of nosocomial pneumonias?

**Self-assessment**    **10 MINUTES**

1. What is the difference between pressure-reducing and pressure-relieving systems?
2. Name two types of each.
3. Why is it important to have a two-way stretch cover on mattresses?

. . . . . . . . . . . . . . . . . . . . . . . . . . . . . . . . .

## FEEDBACK

1. You should have said that pressure-reducing systems increase the surface area in contact with the skin, and pressure-relieving systems move under the body to relieve the pressure on it.
2. For pressure-reducing systems you could have mentioned fibre-filled overlays, foam overlays, foam mattresses, water-filled, air-filled, low air loss and air-fluidised. Pressure-relieving systems include electric air-filled alternating systems and the airwave mattresses.
3. Two-way stretch covers reduce the risk of hammocking for patients, reduce the risk of infection and increase the life span of the mattresses.

. . . . . . . . . . . . . . . . . . . . . . . . . . . . . . . . .

in an organised way and not just using something because one person likes it, or it is on special offer. Price may not be an accurate guide either. What is needed is value for money, reliability and a long life span along with effectiveness.

From the middle of 1998, all equipment has had to bear the European mark, signifying that it has reached a standard of safety, quality and effectiveness accepted throughout Europe. To ensure that this happens, the Medical Devices Agency will work closely with the European Community and manufacturers (O'Dea 1994).

### Paying for equipment

How you pay for your equipment is also of concern, and may depend on the level you are going for. The choices are:

- purchase—outright buying
- lease—for a fixed term
- rental—daily, weekly or monthly rates negotiated according to need.

Table 4.1 shows the advantages and disadvantages of each method.

## 4.2 THE ROLE OF THE CLINICAL NURSE SPECIALIST (CNS)

While clinical nurse specialists are not new, it is only recently that there has been an increase in the number specialising in tissue viability, because of the increasing awareness of problems in this area. These include not only pressure sores, but also wound care in general and leg ulcers, and there are two other

**Table 4.1** Advantages and disadvantages of different methods of paying for equipment

|  | Advantages | Disadvantages |
|---|---|---|
| Purchase | No ongoing costs<br>One-off capital outlay<br>Remains your property<br>Can be purchased with trust funds | Equipment will date<br>Maintenance costs<br>Storage<br>Becomes a capital asset and liable for tax |
| Lease | Reduces capital outlay<br>Equipment can be upgraded<br>Easy to budget<br>Fully maintained by leasing company | Equipment never owned |
| Rental | Product matched to patients' needs<br>Flexibility of choice<br>Maintained by company<br>Removed as soon as use over | Equipment never owned<br>Difficult to budget |

distance learning packs in this series covering these specific issues. There is still much confusion about the role of a clinical nurse specialist, and this subsection discusses this and what the role should entail.

## Problems of the CNS role

Problems related to the role of the CNS are well documented; Sparacino (1986) gives a good overview of many of them. These people often find themselves in a kind of no man's land, with confusion amongst managers, medical staff and other nurses, as to what they should be doing. Williams (1993) looks particularly at the role of the CNS in the community and finds that there are the following problems in performing the role:

- role ambiguity
- the feeling that the CNS deskills other nurses; (this will be looked at further on)
- task orientation
- credibility of the CNS, especially in specialised care settings such as the community.

Sparacino (1986) and Williams (1993) along with others identify the four main components of the CNS role as:

- clinical
- teaching
- management
- research.

A more recent debate that has been added to the arena covers nurses who are increasingly taking on certain aspects of the doctor's role, particularly ones requiring technical skills, and this is being encouraged from a high level in many areas in an attempt to reduce junior doctors' hours (University of Sheffield 1994). A CNS should be a competent nurse with an in-depth knowledge of her speciality, not just a skilled technician. She should work alongside doctors and other members of the team to improve patient care and, if necessary, speak for the patients. A person operating at the true level of a CNS is in an ideal position to bridge the theory/practice gap. A CNS needs to negotiate her job profile with management, and should then expect their support in carrying it out. As far as deskilling other nurses goes, the main role and the most important part of the job is teaching, so she should be passing on her up-to-date knowledge to colleagues, not taking over that area of a patient's care. Credibility has to be established in any area, such are the attitudes of health care workers, and, while it may be desirable to have a special qualification to work in one area, such as the community, this can hardly be expected across the board. The key to acceptance is the personality of the CNS, and the sound knowledge base which allows her to deal with problems in a confident and effective manner.

## The tissue viability CNS

The CNS in tissue viability, unlike some of the other specialities, does not have a specific training. This is presently being looked at by the NATVN who are concerned that anyone can be appointed to the post without specialist knowledge or a clear definition of what the role entails. The role should aim to improve patient care and should include:

- education—to many different people (see p. 56)
- coordinating care—not taking over from staff
- bringing up-to-date research information into practice
- being involved in contracting discussions to provide the service required by the users
- supporting nursing staff in their efforts to improve care, even when this brings them into conflict with other professionals, which can often happen
- moving nursing forward in the field of tissue viability.

All of this requires a resourceful and dynamic personality, not easily deterred by any problems. A book edited by Menard (1987) provides a good overview of some of these areas and issues.

**Activity** 20 MINUTES

Article 6 in the Reader (p. 124) involves a specialist nurse being called in for advice. Having read this, answer the following questions.

1. What advantages did John identify following the involvement of the nurse specialist?
2. Look at the views of the community and research nurses. Then, in the spaces provided below, write notes about John's problems as they were perceived by each of the nurses. Do you notice any difference between them?

**District nurse**

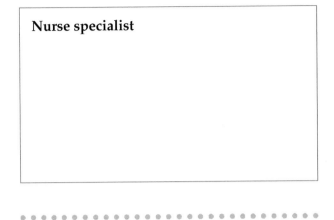

Nurse specialist

## FEEDBACK

1. John was shown what his pressure sore looked like for the first time. It was then explained to him how important his lifting exercises were and, having seen the size of the sore, he was able to relate to the importance of moving. He was also pleased with the new dressings recommended, as they required less frequent dressing changes, which in fact improved his quality of life.
2. The district nurse mentioned general health matters, the inconvenience of the pressure sore, how his family life was restricted by the frequent dressing changes, and John's concern regarding future hospital admissions.

    The research nurse noted how the wound interfered with family life and made John feel he had lost a lot of his privacy and independence, and his dislike of hospital admission. She also did a full wound assessment, noted problems with the wound dressing staying in place, particularly relating to when he was sitting, and the importance of improving his nutrition. She then used her knowledge of recent laboratory studies, and her own experience to select a dressing to meet John's needs. She had a meeting with the district nurse to discuss the changes in care.

This activity should have shown you how a nurse with specialist knowledge can improve the quality of life for a patient, and provide a comprehensive patient assessment relating to her own area but nevertheless encompassing an holistic approach. This is because of her up-to-date knowledge in her own field, enabling her to make an effective treatment plan. She liaised with the district nurse about the change in care, even though her initial visit was to John while in hospital. Although she was fulfilling a clinical role, she taught the patient, the district nurse gained knowledge of new dressings which she would be able to use in the future, and she used knowledge of research and experience on which to base her decisions.

As well as the person herself, the health care team need to accept the CNS for what she is and the knowledge she has if they wish to improve the quality of care and move nursing forward. Additionally they need to help her maximise her time, especially as she may cover a wide area in her work, and before involving her in patient care, make sure that the patient is aware of why she is being involved.

### Activity                    10 MINUTES

Think of a CNS in your area and the role he or she plays. Using the list below, tick off yes or no opposite the statements.

The CNS does the following:

| | | |
|---|---|---|
| 1. Brings in new ideas | Yes | No |
| 2. Provides you with support for decisions made | Yes | No |
| 3. Criticises treatment already in place | Yes | No |
| 4. Helps with obtaining specialist equipment/supplies | Yes | No |
| 5. Takes over the care of the patient | Yes | No |
| 6. Educates staff and patients | Yes | No |
| 7. Provides recent research-based care initiatives | Yes | No |
| 8. Does not like to become clinically involved. | Yes | No |

## FEEDBACK

Your answers may well reflect the working relationship you have with the CNS, or they may be indicators of problems in the working relationship. These can occur from both sides. Look at the next activity, and see how supportive you are of the CNS in his/her role.

### Activity                    10 MINUTES

Consider the ways in which you involve the CNS in the care of your patients by answering the following questions.

- Do you always arrange a joint visit?    Yes    No

- Do you always have the patient ready at the appointment time?    Yes    No

- Do you explain to the patient about the visit?  Yes  No

- Do you only seek advice from the CNS when all else fails?  Yes  No

- Do you consult the CNS before trying any other strategies?  Yes  No

- Do you provide all the clinical details to the CNS?  Yes  No

## FEEDBACK

Have your answers highlighted any areas you feel may hamper the CNS in his/her role?

Making an appointment means fitting patient visits into a busy schedule. There may be the odd occasion when the CNS is unable to arrive on time, but this is often because when arriving at the previous appointment the patient was not ready to be seen, or was unaware that the CNS was going to visit or why. The CNS invariably covers a wide area in her/his role; your visit will only be part of a very busy day. The targets set in relation to home visits have also increased the pressures for all staff working in the community.

Knowing when to call the CNS can be more difficult, but calling him/her out as a first resource is as bad as leaving it so late that by the time he or she is consulted a grade 4 pressure sore has developed. A CNS is in post to help you and your patients, but it needs cooperation from both sides for the system to work effectively.

## 4.3 EDUCATION

Education is identified by many as the key to effective prevention and management of pressure sores (DoH 1993). It needs to include everyone involved in the management and care of patients at risk. The 1995 NHS Executive recommendations include communication as a key strategy, encompassing education to clinicians, and passing on knowledge of successful initiatives to others. This subsection looks at who, how and why to educate.

### Who educates?

Because the whole problem has historically been seen as a nursing problem, educational initiatives, such as they are, have been aimed at nursing staff. Even these were not given high priority, and the first people to provide comprehensive teaching packages were the commercial companies who market equipment and dressings. Some of these were product orientated, some not, but it is a sad indictment of the priority given to understanding this problem that companies took the lead in providing much needed education. Individuals in the tissue viability world set up their own courses, namely Flanagan and Dealey, but it is only very recently that an ENB course (N49) has been recognised. Some teaching options other than courses, either commercially prepared or home-made, are:

- videos
- resource packs
- slides
- study days
- conferences
- classroom teaching
- learning by example.

The last two can be far from ideal, and only increase the theory/practice gap.

Walsh & Ford (1989) recognised that many student nurses are taught about pressure sores in the classroom early on in their training, and then not again. As a result they often pick up ritualistic practice from the wards, and end up knowing how (the how not always being up to date) and not why. Classroom teaching can be done by people who have no recent clinical experience on which to draw and, while they may be up to date with recent research, current practical knowledge may be missing. Wright (1991) and Castledine (1987) feel that clinical nurse specialists should be the key educators, as they can bridge the theory/practice gap, and can include clinical problems in their teaching. They should also be up to date with the latest research. If there is not a CNS, teaching should be done by people with a current clinical role.

### Educating nursing staff

The field of pressure sores is one which has expanded and changed rapidly, with increasing awareness and knowledge as can be seen by the increase in literature since the late 1970s. There are now many different products and dressings on the market, all claiming to be the answer to the problem. Additionally, staff are expected to be aware of some of the aspects already discussed, such as monitoring, grading, and debates going on within the field. If there is a CNS, he or she should have that knowledge, but one person having it is of little use to patients in different care settings. Equally, it is unrealistic to expect all staff to keep up to date in every area of nursing. While nurses with an interest in tissue viability, and pressure sores in particular, can attend study days and incorporate relevant assignments into other courses, such as conversion courses, management courses, etc., this will not solve the problem of spreading information to the majority of people.

A way to overcome this is by creating a link nurse scheme, where dedicated nurses are identified to attend structured teaching sessions, with the result that they become a resource in their own area. As they gain in confidence with their new-found knowledge, the ideal is that they then teach within their own area, but in any case, they certainly feed back at staff meetings following their own sessions. For this system to work, it is essential to have management back-up to enable the nurses to attend study sessions, allow them to provide feedback, and have enough confidence to give them some autonomy to try to change practice at work. Additionally, the person appointed should have an initial interest, and be a permanent member of the ward or team staff. Where a link nurse scheme exists, it is not unusual to find very enthusiastic members of the nurse team, who are glad to have a specific role, providing advice to patients and staff, and compiling educational aids such as notice boards or reading folders, and the increasing awareness having a measurable effect on nursing care. The link nurse should provide the link between nursing staff and the CNS and a two-way communication (see Reader Article 7, p. 127).

**Activity** — **10 MINUTES**

Reader Article 7 describes a link nurse scheme. Read this and then answer the following questions.

1. What are the qualities necessary for a link nurse?
2. What are the benefits of the role?
3. What are the drawbacks of the role?

## FEEDBACK

You should have mentioned the following.

1. A link nurse needs to be keen, enthusiastic and motivated, have a special interest in the subject, and have good presentation and teaching skills.
2. Advantages are said to be improved communication; the potential for improved patient care; relating theory to practice with an improvement in clinical practice.
3. Disadvantages are the problems of time away from patients to attend meetings; possible erosion of the CNS role; lack of incentives for the extra work and responsibility; the problem of new nurses joining an established group.

Other advantages can be meeting nurses from other areas during the study sessions and exchanging ideas; also the constant motivating presence of a link nurse on the ward can prevent backsliding of the change process. Link nurse groups do not have to be solely for link nurses, and other paramedic groups, dietitians, etc. can all benefit from the network. In areas where a network is less practical, such as rural community nursing, it is still possible to have a dedicated nurse for the subject, who attends study days and is given assistance to subscribe to relevant magazines and encouragement to provide feedback to other staff. Providing the opportunity, time and possibly postal finance to provide a newsletter might overcome some of these problems.

## Education of patients and carers

This is a key group for the education process, particularly in the community, where continuous 24-hour nursing care of individual patients is not provided. Included in this group should also be home care workers and NVQ students, who are in fact the people giving the hands-on care and in the best position to notice early signs of pressure damage if they know what they are looking for. While many district nurses provide education on an informal basis for these people, there is seldom time for a more structured approach. Education at this level should include the following.

- Skin care:
  —what to look for as an early sign of pressure damage
  —how to care for skin, what to apply and not apply to it
  —the importance of keeping skin dry.
- Nutrition:
  —its role in pressure sore prevention
  —how to achieve improved nutritional/fluid intake in the individual circumstances.
- Movement:
  —why it is important
  —how it can be achieved in individual circumstances
  —how and why it is important to lift correctly when helping to move patients.
- Equipment:
  —the basics of any equipment being used, especially if it is electrical and in the patient's home
  —how to spot if it is not working properly, and what to do if that is the case.
- Wound—why it smells or leaks and how you hope to manage this.
- Advice—where to get it.

There are specific teaching aids appearing now aimed at this group, such as the Department of Health booklet entitled *Relieving the Pressure* (Reader Article 8, p. 129), and videos. Access to this group can also be gained through organisations such as Share the Care, and in these cases you may pick up people caring for patients at home who are desperate for knowledge but, because they are not involved with any health care professionals, have no way of knowing where to go for advice. Leaflets in doctors' surgeries with local contact numbers may also provide welcome help lines for carers or patients. It is also important to remember that some patients have a greater knowledge of this area in relation to their own care than health professionals, and an article by Baroness Masham (1994; Reader Article 9, p. 140) makes sobering reading on this subject.

## Activity　　20 MINUTES

In Reader Article 6 (p. 124) by Evans & Fear about the patient John, we have already looked at how education to the patient improved his knowledge of his condition, made him more likely to comply with his lifting exercises, because he now understood why they were important, and resulted in a more positive patient outlook. Think of a conscious patient in your area who has or has had a pressure sore of grade 2 or over, then using Table 4.2 identify the areas in which you have educated your patient and or main carer.

| Table 4.2 | | |
| --- | --- | --- |
| | *Patient* | *Carer* |
| Nutrition | Yes/No | Yes/No |
| Movement and its importance | Yes/No | Yes/No |
| Equipment in use and how to check serviceability | Yes/No | Yes/No |
| Wound problems and why occurring | Yes/No | Yes/No |

## FEEDBACK

Has this activity highlighted any pitfalls in your own practice, and do you think you can improve on patient education? If so, write down your findings and discuss them with some of your work colleagues, or discuss obtaining some educational aids for patients.

## Education of medical staff

The absence of input into medical staff training of anything related to wound care or pressure sores is well summed up by Bennett & Moody (1995). When education is given, it is provided by other medical staff, and rarely nurses, yet arguably this is often where the greatest knowledge base now lies. Some medical staff actively encourage a multidisciplinary approach where the expertise of everyone can contribute to patient care, but some remain reluctant to accept that nurses with an interest and specialist knowledge backed up by sound education can contribute to wound management. At the end of this controversy lies the patient who as a result does not always receive the best care. Because all staff do not have the same knowledge base, expensive and inappropriate use of dressings can result, but this is where working together and education would help to solve the problem. The problem of dressing use will be looked at in Section 5.

Medical education is an ideal area for CNS input, particularly to new house officers, or to GPs. The education should include:

- physiology and pathophysiology
- main risk factors
- importance of medical input in relation to nutrition and physiological imbalance
- knowledge of wound healing
- optimum environment for wound healing
- use of modern dressing products.

Common areas of conflict in patient care relate to mobilising patients; medical staff often construe this as sitting out, which has already been shown to be a risk factor. Greater awareness of the pathophysiology and risk factors, combined with liaison with nursing staff, may prevent this and still allow for a patient to be truly mobilised, that is walked on the ward between periods of resting in bed. Passive physiotherapy can also play a role and be taught to carers. An awareness of the importance of nutrition in both wound healing and pressure sore prevention could result in more appropriate alternative methods of feeding for compromised patients, until such time as they can take in normal amounts of food. Other potential areas for conflict between nursing staff and medical staff can be choice of wound dressings and referral to other services.

## Activity　　2–2½ HOURS

Having read this section on the importance of education, and the sections before it, carry out the following.

1. Prepare a 30-minute teaching session for other staff in your area on causes of pressure sores.

Target it at qualified or unqualified staff, and allow 20 minutes for you to talk and 10 minutes for questions and a questionnaire to test their learning.

2. Write down key points that you might put on a transparency for overhead projection or in a handout for staff.

3. Devise a questionnaire to give to the staff to test what they have learnt from the session.

## FEEDBACK

Your lesson should cover all the topics discussed in this section, and what staff who have access to study days or educational sessions such as this should be doing to spread their knowledge to as many other staff as possible, and not keep it to themselves. Boxes 4.2 and 4.3 give suggestions for lesson content and questions. Try, if you can, to carry out the teaching exercise and questionnaire; you may be pleasantly surprised by the response.

### Educating other areas/personnel

Also to be included in an education programme should be:

- paramedics—including physiotherapists, occupational therapists, ambulance personnel
- purchasers
- education on publishing in journals, to share knowledge and initiatives with health professionals in other areas.

---

**Box 4.3** Questionnaire

**Unqualified staff**
What is the difference between intrinsic and extrinsic factors?

What are the main principles of skin care?

Why is nutrition important in pressure sore prevention?

What is your role in pressure sore prevention?

**Qualified staff**
What is the effect of pressure and shear forces on the tissues?

What are the effects of:

1. intrinsic
2. extrinsic

factors on the body?

What is the main role of risk assessment tools?

Who should receive education on pressure sore prevention?

---

**Self-assessment**     20 MINUTES

1. Suggest five groups of people who should receive education in relation to pressure sores.
2. Who would be an appropriate person to educate such groups?
3. Suggest at least five ways in which education could be delivered.

---

**Box 4.2** Lesson plan

**Unqualified staff**

| | |
|---|---|
| Intrinsic and extrinsic factors—which are which | 5 minutes |
| Skin care and reporting changes to qualified staff | 7 minutes |
| Importance of correct lifting and handling | 5 minutes |
| Importance of nutrition and feeding patients and how to overcome problems | 7 minutes |

Stress their role in reporting back to qualified staff changes in skin condition and non-compliance of patients.

**Qualified staff**
Overview of effect of pressure and shear on skin and tissues

+

| | |
|---|---|
| Intrinsic and extrinsic factors and how they affect tissues | 15 minutes |
| Risk assessment and its place as an indicator of risk | 5 minutes |
| Importance of education and multidisciplinary approach | 5 minutes |

Make sure that they understand:

- how damage occurs and the effect it has on tissues
- factors that increase risk
- use of risk assessment tools
- importance of education—particularly to patients.

## FEEDBACK

1. You should have included all of the following in your answer:

   - nursing staff
   - medical staff
   - patients and carers—relatives and unqualified staff
   - paramedics
   - purchasers.

2. The ideal person to educate is a clinical nurse specialist or someone with current clinical input.

3. Education can be delivered in the following ways:

   - study days
   - link nurse groups
   - videos
   - leaflets
   - resource packs
   - slides
   - classroom teaching
   - by example.

## 4.4 DISCHARGE PLANNING

With the change in emphasis in health care from secondary to primary care, many patients who would previously have been kept in hospital are being discharged into the community or private sector. Among this group are patients with pressure sores or at high risk of developing them. If discharge is not planned, major problems can result. This can also increase community costs. A survey in Lincoln (Preston 1991) found that the biggest cost factor in caring for patients with pressure sores was district nurse time. Community resources are scarce and often insufficient time is given to arranging a package of care for discharge. The district nurse, clinical nurse specialist or discharge liaison nurse should be involved in planning sooner rather than later.

Without a doubt, communication is the key to success and yet this simple action is so often overlooked. Each care setting needs to be aware of problems encountered by the other side. Hospital staff may be under great pressure from the medical staff or the patient to bring about a speedy discharge, even if this is not what they feel is best for the patient. The bed may be needed, particularly on an acute ward. In the community, private sector and community hospitals, resources will undoubtedly be stretched as the money for primary care initiatives has not been forthcoming; funds given to social services are intended for social not health needs. This is looked at in more detail in Section 8. Main problems in discharge arrangements which can cause difficulties for the patient and community staff are:

- Lack of reassessment (this can be by hospital staff before patients go home, or by community staff following patient transfer) resulting in incorrect use of resources. Typically patients who have been allocated a high level of equipment on admission to hospital remain on this to the end of their stay, even when it is no longer necessary.
- Failure to notify primary care staff.
- Leaving it too late to inform community staff for resources to be obtained.
- Lack of understanding by hospital staff of limited community resources.
- Lack of resources in community and private sectors.
- Lack of knowledge of home circumstances and ability of carer, if any.
- Inappropriate community placement by social services staff.

Again, education of the personnel involved is the key. Additionally there should be policies which cover all areas, and promote seamless care. A discharge flow chart such as the one shown in Figure 4.1 can be used to help staff and increase their awareness of community problems. There will always be occasions when the unforeseen happens, but if in these cases more direct communication were made, much bad feeling would be avoided. If the patient will be new to the district nurse caseload, or if there are complex problems with wound care, the district nurse may like to visit the patient in hospital to discuss the care with ward staff, and equally nursing and residential care managers may like this option. It may not always be taken up, but at least the option should be there.

### Activity — 20 MINUTES

Article 10 in the Reader (p. 142) looks at discharge into the community and is useful because it pulls together many of the key points mentioned in the education and equipment sections. Read this article, then look at Case history 2 and identify the factors which contributed to the development of a pressure sore for Mrs Smith.

## FEEDBACK

You should have identified the following factors:

- Lack of referral to the district nurse by hospital staff, despite the fact that this was obviously a patient at risk. This also shows ignorance by nursing staff of the fact that patients in residential

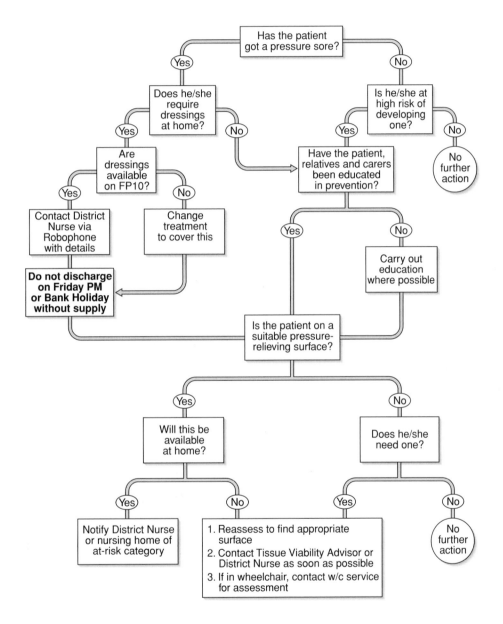

**Fig. 4.1** Discharge flow chart.

care do not receive nursing input except from the district nurse.

- Lack of provision of education to the care assistant on basic causes and risks of pressure sore development.
- Lack of understanding by residential home managers of risks and need to seek help earlier.
- Lack of risk assessment before the district nurse was involved. This included the fact that the hospital staff had obviously not assessed and warned the residential staff of the risk, and the residential staff had not assessed the patient at transfer.

As this history states, the resultant costs were in money and suffering to the patient, and in this case avoidable.

● ● ● ● ● ● ● ● ● ● ● ● ● ● ● ● ● ● ● ● ● ● ● ● ● ● ● ● ● ● ●

## Activity                          10 MINUTES

Think of a patient in your own area who is at risk and is about to be or has just been discharged, and answer the following questions.

1. Has the patient been assessed for the change of care setting and in his/her present condition?
2. Has the district nurse or private sector manager been informed of the discharge and risk category?
3. Were/are the hospital nursing staff aware of the home and social circumstances?
4. Has education been provided to all carers concerned?
5. Is suitable equipment available for the patient if relevant?

If you answer 'No' to any of the above, list the steps you can take to put the matter right.

● ● ● ● ● ● ● ● ● ● ● ● ● ● ● ● ● ● ● ● ● ● ● ● ● ● ● ● ● ● ●

## FEEDBACK

If the answers are all positive, this is a good sign for your patients; if not, has the exercise shown you some areas which could be improved?

If you are in the community setting, what do you intend to do about improving the situation? A working group, or getting representation on a policy group would help. Could you arrange to talk to groups of nurses from the hospitals, for example link nurses, to raise their awareness of the problems? If really necessary, start to liaise with wards and managers after problem discharges, rather than just coping, to let them know the problems involved.

● ● ● ● ● ● ● ● ● ● ● ● ● ● ● ● ● ● ● ● ● ● ● ● ● ● ● ● ● ● ●

One way around the problem that has been adopted by some areas is the appointment of a discharge liaison nurse, and also liaison can be part of the role of the CNS. However, they cannot check every discharge, and it is essential that all staff take responsibility for ensuring that care of patients continues beyond their own care setting.

As already mentioned, a major problem in the community is lack of resources. Although some areas have community loan stores, these are often poorly run in terms of supplying equipment quickly to patients, and do not have enough equipment in stock. Some areas are beginning to tackle this, having put up a case of need for more resources, but the problem is compounded by the fact that social services hold the purse strings for community care, but are meant to provide equipment for patients based on social rather than nursing need. Until money begins to follow patients, there will be problems.

## Self-assessment                   10 MINUTES

List five measures which would help to facilitate better discharge for patients.

● ● ● ● ● ● ● ● ● ● ● ● ● ● ● ● ● ● ● ● ● ● ● ● ● ● ● ● ● ● ●

## FEEDBACK

You should have identified the following:

- cross-border policy making staff aware of problems in each care setting
- discharge flow chart
- up-to-date patient assessment
- education
- discharge liaison nurse
- improved cross-border relationships and communication.

● ● ● ● ● ● ● ● ● ● ● ● ● ● ● ● ● ● ● ● ● ● ● ● ● ● ● ● ● ● ●

## 4.5 MULTIDISCIPLINARY APPROACH AND FORMATION OF A POLICY

Although the problem of pressure sores remains largely in the nursing domain, there is increasing awareness of the importance of a multidisciplinary approach to tackling the problem. Who exactly is involved will depend to some extent on the care setting, but there is no reason why every area including the private sector cannot provide a team to look at the problem. With the shift to primary care, the ideal would be to have a policy compiled across care boundaries, so that where possible, a common language was being spoken by all staff involved in patient care, for example relating to equipment in use or when grading pressure sores. Examples of personnel who could be involved in groups are:

- Dietitian, to assist with nutritional advice to patients and staff on an individual basis.
- Medical staff—this could include consultants and/or general practitioners, so that they understand the importance of their role in providing medical back-up for conditions predisposing to pressure sores, such as anaemia, and for them to involve other staff in discussions relating to wound care. Also, interested medical staff can help to smooth the path where there is opposition to aspects of pressure sore prevention from colleagues, for example reluctance to involve other health care workers in care of a patient.
- Paramedics such as occupational therapists and physiotherapists, who are often involved in trying to return patients to the home environment and rehabilitate them after illness.
- Social services—often involved in providing equipment for patients in their own homes, and need to liaise with nurse colleagues.
- Medical physics—responsible for maintaining purchased equipment.
- Carers, either social services or the patient's own, although it may take some courage to include the latter group, as they may bring a new perspective to the problem.
- Appropriate nursing staff, such as link nurses, team leaders, community staff.
- Staff from specialist areas such as radiography or intensive care.
- A manager who will probably control the purse strings.

Although all these people have been mentioned, they may not all be needed in every instance, and it should be remembered that large groups with the potential for more disagreement can often take longer to achieve results than small ones. For this reason, sub-groups or working parties may be a more effective way of completing designated work.

## Self-assessment    15 MINUTES

Think of a patient in your care who has a grade 3 or over pressure sore, and list the people involved in his/her care. Then write down anyone else who you think should have been involved but is not.

## FEEDBACK

Your answer will depend on where you are, but you may well have identified some people you feel should have been involved but were not. If so, think about how you may involve them in future cases.

The most important aspect at the beginning is that the group know the size of the pressure sore problem for their area and can set objectives and compile a policy to deal with it. As well as measurable indicators of the problem, a brainstorming session can often identify other important issues which can be addressed by the group. This can be invaluable as staff in different care settings are not always aware of problems encountered outside their own areas.

Some initiatives which can be undertaken by the group are:

- equipment survey, to sort out what is available and in what state it is
- making a business case to finance new equipment
- looking at special areas such as theatre and accident and emergency
- wheelchair survey
- guidelines for pressure sore prevention and management
- education programmes
- auditing effectiveness of measures taken
- inclusion of ambulance personnel
- discharge policy.

The inclusion of the ambulance personnel in a prevention strategy is important, as apart from emergency patients, where increased awareness of patients at risk can enable them to notify casualty to have a pressure-relieving surface available, they can also provide a safer environment for at-risk patients being transferred by ambulance (McClemont et al 1991).

## Implementing a policy

While writing a policy takes time and effort by a few people, the real effort is in ensuring that it does not then sit on shelves unused. It should be user-friendly, with easily identified sections for quick reference. A loose-leaf presentation allows for alterations to be made and ideally the policy should be updated and reviewed every 2 years, especially the areas covering equipment and dressings, where the market and research is constantly changing. One example is the North Lincolnshire Pressure Sore Policy (1993) and another is described in a paper by Moody et al (1992) presented at the First European Conference on Advances in Wound Management.

## Activity    45 MINUTES

Circle 'Yes' or 'No' in relation to your own areas in response to the questions in Table 4.3. If you answer yes to any question marked with an asterisk, give more details.

**Table 4.3**

| Question | Answer | Details |
|---|---|---|
| Do you have a pressure sore policy in place? | Yes/No | |
| Do you know the size of the problem in your area?* | Yes/No | |
| Do you know the equipment resources available to you?* | Yes/No | |
| Do you know who to contact for advice if needed?* | Yes/No | |
| Do you have an education booklet for patients/carers? | Yes/No | |
| If you have a policy, does it cross care boundaries? | Yes/No | |
| Do you have access to a dietitian? | Yes/No | |
| Are you aware of any auditing methods in use relating to pressure sore prevention?* | Yes/No | |

## FEEDBACK

Completing this table may have shown that your area is well down the path to tackling the pressure sore problem, part of the way there, or still with some work to do. Some of the initiatives you could consider, depending on your own area, could be:

- a small prevalence study to indicate the size of the problem
- an equipment survey, to highlight shortfalls
- identification of members who could start a group
- costing of an individual case to show how expensive the problem is
- devising information leaflets for staff relating to some of the issues, e.g. where to access the dietitian, list of equipment available, etc.
- devising a patient information leaflet.

### Selling the policy

Having a policy launch day is a good way of raising awareness and answering any queries. It is more likely to be supported by a wider audience than just nursing staff if all members of the group attend the day and target their own professional colleagues.

Also commercial companies might be asked to sponsor and exhibit if you are endorsing their products. They will be able to show staff the products and discuss usage with them. The day also gives staff a chance to familiarise themselves with the policy content.

Having launched the policy, it is also important to keep staff up to date with progress, for example feeding back results of any prevalence or incidence data obtained, particularly if they show a reduction in the size of the problem. You should also involve staff in audits of areas of the policy. That way they are more likely to take ownership of the policy and work towards its success.

**Self-assessment**　　　20 MINUTES

Identify five key points to help in the success of a pressure sore prevention policy.

## FEEDBACK

You should have identified the following:

- multidisciplinary group involvement
- awareness of the main problem areas and the size of the problem

- user-friendly style
- applicable across care boundaries
- involvement of all staff in policy launch.

• • • • • • • • • • • • • • • • • • • • • • • • • • • • • • • • • • •

If you have a policy but are doubtful of its effectiveness, you may now be able to identify where there are problems. If you do not have a policy, this may set you on the road to starting one.

## SUMMARY

Having studied this section on prevention of pressure sores, which should always be the key aim of any programme, you should now have a greater knowledge of the many ways to work towards this, including the following.

- How to choose equipment which is best suited to your patients and their needs, and the staff training necessary for this.

- The key role which can be taken by the clinical nurse specialist in prevention of pressure sores.

- An education programme is essential and needs to include patients and carers as well as all health care workers.

- Communication and early discharge planning are important in providing quality care and preventing pressure sores occurring after discharge.

- Setting up a multidisciplinary policy is an essential part of providing cohesive prevention and management strategies.

REFERENCES

Bennett G, Moody M 1995 Wound care for health professionals. Chapman & Hall, London

Castledine G 1987 The development of the C.N.S. in the U.K. Acta Hospitalia 27(3): 67–79

Dealey C 1995 Mattresses and beds. Journal of Wound Care 4(9): 409–412

Department of Health 1993 Pressures sores; a key quality indicator. DoH, Lancashire

Masham (Baroness) 1994 Healing: a patient's perspective. Journal of Wound Care 3(4): 195–196

McClemont E, Woodcock N, Oliver S, Hinton C, Preston K, Phillips J 1991 Journal of Tissue Viability 2(4): 114–117

Menard S (ed) 1987 The clinical nurse specialist: perspectives on practice. John Wiley, Canada

Moody M, Nichols R, Robertson J, Swain I. 1992 Developing a pressure sore prevention and management policy. In: Harding K, Leaper D, Turner T (eds) First European Conference on Advances in Wound Management. Macmillan Magazines, London

NHS Executive 1995 Pressure sores, using information. NHS Executive, Leeds

North Lincolnshire Pressure Sore Policy 1993 Prevention and management of pressure damage. North Lincolnshire Health Authority, Lincolnshire

O'Dea K 1994 The problem for equipment manufacturers in developing clinical research. Journal of Tissue Viability 4(3): 79–83

Preston K 1991 Counting the cost of pressure sores. Community Outlook 1(9): 19–24

Ryan D 1983 The influence of environmental temperature on catabolism using the clinitron air fluidised bed. Intensive Care Medicine 9: 279–281

Sparacino P 1986 The clinical nurse specialist. Nursing Practice 1: 215–228

University of Sheffield 1994 Reduction of junior doctors' hours in Trent Region: the nursing contribution. NHS Executive, Sheffield

Walsh M, Ford P 1989 Nursing rituals, research and rational action. Heinemann Nursing, Oxford

Williams A 1993 Steps to develop a working relationship: an evaluation of the community-based clinical nurse specialist. Professional Nurse (Sept): 806–812

Wright S 1991 The nurse as a consultant. Nursing Standard 5(20): 31–34

Young J 1992 The use of specialised beds and mattresses. Journal of Tissue Viability 2(3): 79–81

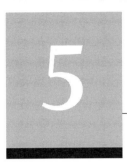

# 5 Treatment and management of pressure sores

So far we have looked at how pressure sores occur, ways of identifying people at risk, and how to prevent pressure sores, but the reality is that they still happen. The next step is to look at how to manage pressure sores when they do develop.

## LEARNING OUTCOMES

At the end of this section, you will be able to:

- describe the process of wound healing
- list the factors which delay and assist this process
- explain how to plan appropriate care for patients with pressure sores.

## 5.1 PHYSIOLOGY OF WOUND HEALING

Despite the fact that nurses are frequently at the forefront of wound management, their knowledge of the physiology of wound healing is often poor. Dealey (1994a) gives three reasons why nurses should have this knowledge:

- knowing the normal physiology enables them to recognise when something abnormal is occurring
- knowing the stages of wound healing helps in the selection of appropriate dressings
- knowing the nutritional requirements of the stages of the wound healing process enables the nurse to ensure adequate dietary intake.

There are two main types of wound healing:

- by primary intention, where the two edges are drawn together as in surgical wounds
- by secondary intention, where the wound heals by filling in an area of tissue loss, as in leg ulcers or pressure sores.

### The process of wound healing

Wound healing occurs in three stages; some people split the second stage into two to give four stages, but the process is the same. The stages are:

- inflammation
- proliferation
- maturation.

A brief summary follows. For more detail it is suggested that you read a textbook on wound healing and/or some of the references provided.

The stages of wound healing last for varying overlapping periods, dependent on the type, size and position of the wound and factors which may enhance or delay wound healing.

### Inflammation

This stage protects the body from further damage and starts to deal with toxins and kill bacteria. Neutrophils and monocytes are produced in increasing numbers and start ingesting foreign material, the process known as phagocytosis. Some monocytes mature into macrophages which continue phagocytosis as well as storing debris and stimulating antibody production. They also release enzymes which help to prolong the inflammatory stage as necessary, using a feedback mechanism (Bennett & Moody 1995). The wound lacks any tensile strength at this stage, which can last from 0–4 days. If for any reason the inflammatory stage does not occur, or has its effect reduced, wounds are unlikely to heal. Wounds at this stage of healing are vascular, with surrounding heat and redness to the wound.

### Proliferation

This is the stage where the wound begins to replace lost tissue. Collagen fibres begin to form, and it is this which gives strength to the wound, but at this early stage the fibres are not laid down in an organised way, so their effect is reduced. They do support the capillary loops and new fragile capillary buds—the base for formation of granulation tissue across the wound—whose formation has been promoted by the macrophages. This process is known as angiogenesis and promotes the increased supply of oxygen to the wound, speeding up the healing process. Epithelial cells can then begin to migrate across the wound surface. To do this they need a moist environment and viable granulation tissue. Wounds that are granulating have a shiny bright red surface and are quite moist (see Plate 10, between pp. 22 and 23). As epithelialisation occurs, the wound becomes a paler pink, and is less moist.

## Maturation

This is the period when structure and function are returned to the wound (Bennett & Moody 1995). The collagen fibres start to rearrange themselves into a more organised structure, increasing the tensile strength of the wound. This can take up to 1 year, and even then the wound site will not regain the same strength as previously. This is why it is so important to continue to protect newly healed pressure sores. This is the stage when the skin heals over and scarring occurs. Look at Figure 3 in Reader Article 11 (p. 145) where a wound shows granulation tissue in the centre, epithelialisation at the edge of the open area, and maturation of the surrounding border. It can also be seen that this tissue is still fragile and would damage again easily. It has taken 3 months to reach this stage.

**Self-assessment**    20 MINUTES

1. Listed below are the three stages of wound healing. Opposite each one write down the main function of that stage.

   Inflammation:

   Proliferation:

   Maturation:

2. What is angiogenesis?
3. What role do macrophages play in wound healing?

## FEEDBACK

1. You should have said that the inflammatory stage protects the body from further damage, the proliferative stage replaces lost tissue volume, and the maturation stage restores function and strength to the tissues, although not at the original level.
2. Angiogenesis is the promotion of new capillary formation by macrophages which helps to bring oxygen to the wound.
3. Apart from this, macrophages ingest debris, stimulate antibody production and release enzymes to prolong the inflammatory stage if necessary.

This is a very brief overview of the healing process, but anyone dealing with wounds should know what is occurring if they are to accurately assess what stage the wound is at and what dressings should be used.

**Activity**    10 MINUTES

Choose one patient in your area with a wound; it does not have to be a pressure sore. Now answer the following questions.

1. Is the wound healing by secondary or primary intention?
2. Which stage of the healing process is it at? Give a reason for your answer.

## FEEDBACK

Your answers will depend on patient chosen.

1. If you have chosen a patient with an open wound, it is healing by secondary intention; if a sutured wound, it is healing by primary intention.
2. With a sutured wound you would only be able to tell if it was in the inflammatory stage, when the wound would be warm and with some redness and slight swelling adjacent to it. If the wound is healing by secondary intention, you should have based your choice on its appearance and the time since it appeared. This may have highlighted some problems for you if the wound has been long-standing and not progressed. This is because there are other factors that affect wound healing, which we will look at in Section 5.2. Additionally the wound may contain slough or necrotic tissue with the result that you could not identify a healing process, as you would be unable to see the tissue in the wound. This too will be looked at in Section 5.2. Slough is dead tissue and fibrin fibres, and needs to be removed from the wound for healing to occur; it forms a yellow film of varying thickness over wounds. Necrotic tissue is the same except that it has been exposed to the air, so that it takes on a hard leathery, black appearance.

## 5.2 THE HEALING ENVIRONMENT

Knowing the physiology of wound healing is important, but in the author's experience many medical and nursing staff expect a wound to heal because it has a certain dressing on it, or because pressure relief is being provided. They are amazed when this does not happen, and yet many local and systemic factors will affect wound healing, so it is essential to have a knowledge of these.

## Local factors

These relate to factors at the wound site and a complete list is given in Section 5.5 which looks at dressings. However, three of the main ones are:

- maintaining a moist environment by use of a suitable dressing (see Sect. 5.5 for reasons behind this and how to achieve it)
- freedom of the wound from any form of contamination—this could include foreign bodies such as gauze fibres, stitches, or slough, and also chemicals in the form of inappropriate use of antiseptics (see Sect. 5.5)
- removal of pressure from the wound in the case of a pressure sore.

## Systemic factors

These are factors relating to the patient's general condition which affect wound healing, and if these are not addressed in the treatment plan, it is totally unrealistic to expect wound healing to occur, and indeed there may be further tissue breakdown. Systemic factors include the following.

- Nutrition—the two essentials are protein, as without this rebuilding of the wound and formation of the collagen fibres will not occur, and energy, as tissue repair greatly increases cellular activity and insufficient energy intake will result in breakdown of body tissue to try to meet the need. Protein is also lost in the wound exudate, and it is important to replace this as well as provide for recommended daily intake. Other elements also play their part in the healing process. Article 2 in the Reader (p. 109) provides an easily readable summary of the key role of certain nutrients in wound healing.

**Activity**                    30 MINUTES

Read Article 2 then answer the following questions. What role do the following play in wound healing?

1. zinc
2. protein
3. glucose
4. vitamin C
5. vitamin E.

## FEEDBACK

You should have said:

1. Zinc—necessary for the action of RNA to promote protein synthesis and collagen formation, which give the wound its strength. In addition, a deficiency reduces the rate of epithelialisation.
2. Protein—an essential nutrient, providing the greater part of the energy requirement for wound healing. To avoid depletion and provide enough, it is necessary to increase the daily intake.
3. Glucose—a primary fuel for tissue repair, needed to meet the increased metabolic need generated by wound healing. Helps preserve the body's protein, as deficiency in glucose results in conversion of protein stocks to supply glucose.
4. Vitamin C—essential for the synthesis of collagen, and deficiency causes capillary fragility. Wounds which have healed may even break down again if sufficient intake is not maintained.
5. Vitamin E—affects the survival of red and white blood cells, and enhances the immune response.

Other systemic factors include:

- Reduced oxygen supply to the wound. In the initial stage of wound healing tissue oxygen is low, but if this level is not raised, cells cannot begin to work and carry out their function, and collagen cannot be synthesised. Factors contributing to this are:
  —anaemia
  —peripheral vascular disease
  —hypotension
  —smoking; smokers also have vitamin deficiencies, particularly vitamin C
  —any factors affecting blood circulation, e.g. cardiac or pulmonary function.
- Anything which affects the stages of wound healing, including:
  —steroids, which reduce the inflammatory stage
  —other anti-inflammatory drugs
  —nutrition, as already shown
  —cytotoxic therapy, which affects cell division.
- The patient's general condition.
- Age, where there is often the combination of decreased nutritional intake, and the fact that cellular activity slows down.
- Diabetes—glycosuria reduces the inflammatory response, and thus the numbers of phagocytic cells present in the wound, resulting in increased risk of infection because of reduced phagocytosis, which delays wound healing.

- Malignancy, which can affect nutritional intake and also increase the metabolic rate without the added factor of a healing wound.
- Incontinence, urinary and faecal, which may cause contamination of the wound depending on where it is situated.

There are also social factors:

- A poor or dirty environment, which may encourage wound infection.
- Financial hardship, which may result in poor nutritional intake.
- Poor patient compliance, particularly if the patient has a pressure sore, and continues to put weight on it, or is unwilling to reduce his or her smoking.

## Activity    1½ HOURS

Article 11 in the Reader (p. 144) is a good case study of a patient with a wound and several problems relating to wound healing. Having read the article, and in conjunction with the text in this section, answer the following questions.

1. List all the factors relating to Mark which could delay wound healing, and state opposite each one why it would delay healing. Example: anaemia—reduces oxygen-carrying capacity of the blood.
2. Choose a patient in your own area who has a wound which is not healing as fast as you would expect. Look at the local and systemic factors, using the nursing and medical notes as well as your nursing knowledge of the patient, then write down any factors which you consider are delaying wound healing for this patient. If you have identified any which have an adverse effect on wound healing, is there anything you can now do to remedy the situation?

## FEEDBACK

1. You should have identified the following factors for Mark:

    - anaemia as quoted
    - general health—condition poor, renal function impaired, which will affect the whole blood chemistry, additionally frequent urinary tract infections which contribute to incontinence and wound contamination
    - slough on the wound, which delays healing until removed

- nutritional intake and loss of protein through the wound
- faecal incontinence causing wound contamination.

2. The response relating to your own patient will vary but you may have identified some factors you were unaware of in relation to wound healing, such as diabetes, anaemia or other systemic factors, or there may be things such as incontinence. Problems relating to nursing such as incontinence, poor nutrition or slough on the wound could be addressed by nursing staff. If there is a more systemic factor, make sure that the doctor is aware of it, so that medical intervention can be arranged.

## Developments in wound care techniques

There are now various ways in which the healing process can be enhanced, some well tried and tested, and some in the early stages of development. Some of these are explained below.

### Specialised mattresses

These are some of the ones already mentioned in the section on pressure-relieving systems (pp. 51–52), but with additional activity said to promote healing. Again, some have documented proof sources, others do not. Examples of relevant literature include Dealey (1994b) looking at the Nimbus II mattress, Lowthian (1995) the Pegasus Airwave mattress, and Ryan (1990) the Clinitron air-fluidised bed.

**Alternating pressure systems.** These all claim some benefit in wound healing, although they have different cycle times and different numbers of cells inflated at any one time. Certainly the relief of pressure helps with wound healing in the case of pressure sores, providing all other factors are considered as well. Different companies advocate use for differing grades of sores, not always with clinical sources to back up their recommendations.

**The airwave systems**: an alternating pressure system. With their very high pressures followed by very low pressures, these use the theory of flushing hyperaemia as an active factor in healing, so that the rapid return of oxygen and nutrients to the wound following the release of the high pressure stage actually speeds up the healing process. Several case histories appear to demonstrate the effectiveness of these systems, for example that of Rithalia (1994; Reader Article 12, p. 147). These are recommended for grade 4 and all other sores.

**Low air loss systems.** With the whole mattress systems incorporated into beds, these are likely to be more effective for wound healing than mattress toppers, again because of the low pressures, and particularly because they can be individually adjusted for patients.

**Air-fluidised systems.** Their main role is for wound healing rather than pressure sore prevention and, although expensive, this needs to be offset against total wound healing time if in fact this is shortened by use of these systems. Some of the properties these unique systems bring to wound healing are protein sparing, where protein is being lost through wound exudate, reduction in catabolic state and stress for the patient, reduction in pain, and a clean environment. Article 11 in the Reader (p. 144) describes why one of these beds was chosen to help in dealing with a patient's wound.

## Growth factors

These were actually recognised over 20 years ago, and are essential for cell proliferation (Cox 1993). They are naturally occurring proteins, and they contribute towards coordinating cell reactions which occur during wound healing. Different growth factors have an effect on different stages of wound healing. Results from clinical trials where growth factors are introduced into chronic wounds are encouraging, and this may be a way forward in the future.

## Hyperbaric oxygen

This is mainly used for necrotising infections in the wound care field, but can also have a role in long-standing problem wounds. It stops the production of some toxins which can cause major tissue problems for patients.

## Lasers

Low power laser therapy is the method of applying light to injuries to stimulate wound healing, the main function being to speed the healing process. Training in its use needs to be given and there are patients for whom use of lasers is contraindicated; however, their use is increasing and there is evidence of their success with various types of wound (James 1995). They can be used by nursing staff.

## Debridement

The fact that slough and necrotic tissue need to be removed before healing can occur has been mentioned, but there are in fact three accepted ways to do this.

- Autolysis, which means rehydrating the tissue, so that the devitalised tissue lifts away from the

wound. This is achieved by encouraging a moist environment at the wound surface.
- Chemical, where the chemical action starts to break down and loosen the dead tissue.
- Surgical, which is without doubt the quickest, but needs weighing up in terms of patient benefits. It can be done under anaesthetic, which in itself carries certain risks, or it can be done on the ward. This will largely depend on the type and size of wound.

## Surgery

Apart from debridement of pressure sores, an operation can be done to cover the sore with a flap of skin and tissue from a suitable site, for example skin and tissue from the buttock can be excised and rotated to cover a deep sacral sore. The flap is then sutured to allow healing to take place. Blood supply is maintained as the flap is not wholly excised and donor sites heal by secondary intention. This is a quicker system, particularly for large sores. However, because of conflicting demands at work, some plastic surgeons can only accept a specific number of patients for this type of surgery and then only after full assessment which includes likely long-term outcomes, and after care arrangements. It is not good use of resources to undertake this surgery on patients who are likely to return to the same environment as before and redevelop a pressure sore.

**Self-assessment** 15 MINUTES

1. Which special mattresses are said to affect healing? How, and for what grade of sores?
2. What are the three ways of carrying out wound debridement?
3. Which systemic factors affect wound healing?

## FEEDBACK

1. You should have said that the following mattresses are said to have an effect on wound healing:

- alternating pressure, by relieving the pressure
- airwave, where the flushing hyperaemia which follows the removal of the high pressure in the mattress' cycle, brings nutrients and oxygen to the wound—grade 4 and under sores
- low air loss, particularly the whole bed systems where the low pressures aid healing—grade 4 and under sores

- air-fluidised, which are protein sparing, reduce stress and the effects of the catabolic state, and provide a clean environment—grade 4 and under sores.

2. Wound debridement can be done by: autolysis, chemical means and surgery.

3. The following systemic factors affect wound healing:

   - nutrition
   - reduced oxygen supply for whatever reason
   - anything which affects the stages of wound healing, such as drugs
   - the patient's general condition
   - social factors.

This subsection should have made you far more aware of the importance of looking at the whole patient in relation to wound healing, and not just relying on dressings and mattresses to achieve miracles. Also you should now know that this field of medicine is not standing still and advances may be just around the corner to improve matters. It may also make you aware of the need to be realistic when planning care, and accept that wound healing may not be achieved in some patients.

## 5.3 INFECTED OR COLONISED?

Despite the fact that there are now problems with antibiotic-resistant infections (Perry 1996) nurses continue to see examples of unnecessary prescribing. The problem is in identifying pressure sores which are infected as against those which are colonised. Pressure sores are not sterile wounds, and the likelihood of obtaining a sterile swab from one is not high, apart from the fact that swabs only identify surface microorganisms. A wound biopsy will identify the true source of infection, but is not a practical option in many cases, because it requires medical staff to carry it out, and there is a cost involved, which would only be justified in cases of long-term unresolved infections. Pressure sores will contain normal flora and some bacteria, such as *Staphylococcus aureus* and *Escherichia coli*, which are found inside the body. This is known as colonisation, and at this level the body can cope with the bacteria. Problems arise when the bacteria reach a level where they compete with the macrophages for nutrients and oxygen from the wound, and tissue reaction starts to occur (Smith & Nephew & RCN 1991). This is known as infection. It is only when the signs of infection appear that you should start to take wound swabs and give systemic antibiotics.

## Identifying the signs of infection

Cutting & Harding (1994) discuss criteria for identifying infection. They list the traditional criteria as:

- abscess, a collection of necrotic tissue and bacteria with some white cells forming pus
- cellulitis, where bacterial infection has caused inflammation of the skin and subcutaneous tissue
- discharge, particularly pus, although other types of fluid may drain with concurrent inflammation.

However, they go on to point out that other factors can indicate infection, and should be watched out for. Not all of them may be present, but these are ones to look out for:

- Delayed healing, which cannot be attributed to some of the factors we have already looked at in Section 5.2.
- Discoloration—and this is where knowledge of normal wound healing and what wounds should look like at the different stages comes in. If the wound appears abnormal, for example dull instead of shiny, and maybe with patches of a different colour, it may be infected; in the case of pseudomonas infection the wound takes on a characteristic green colour.
- Friable granulation tissue, that is it bleeds easily, and the wound can appear raw and red.
- Pain—for example deep pressure sores do not usually hurt much, because the nerve endings which are in the dermis have been destroyed, but new or unexpected pain at the site of the sore is indicative of infection.
- Pocketing or bridging of a wound is usually caused by islands of bacteria preventing overall healing.
- Smell—it would be necessary to have some of the other signs as well before using this as a diagnosis of infection. It is probably true to say that all wounds that are infected smell, but all wounds that smell are not infected. Necrotic, sloughy wounds smell, but are not always infected. Experienced nurses may also be able to recognise different smells, as sloughy wounds smell different from infected wounds, and indeed some infections have a different smell from others.
- Wound breakdown, particularly following apparent healing.
- Pyrexia is another indicator of infection, although you need to know that the patient does not have a urinary or chest infection which may account for the temperature.

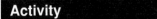

**Activity**      15 MINUTES

Think of a patient in your caseload who is on antibiotics for any type of wound infection. Using Table 5.1, tick off the factors that contributed to the conclusion that the wound was infected and needed antibiotics.

| Table 5.1 | |
| --- | --- |
| *Indicator* | *Present* |
| Abscess | |
| Cellulitis | |
| Discharge | |
| Delayed healing | |
| Discoloration | |
| Friable granulation tissue | |
| Pain | |
| Pocketing or bridging of the wound | |
| Smell | |
| Wound breakdown | |
| Pyrexia | |

## FEEDBACK

You may have been able to tick off several, but often the only factor is smell because a wound is sloughy, and this is not enough to indicate an infected wound. Even if you took a wound swab which came back positive, you probably now realise that this may only have identified microorganisms which are colonising the wound, not ones which are infecting it, and your patient may be receiving unnecessary antibiotic therapy.

Deciding that a wound is infected needs observation and knowledge, particularly if overprescribing of antibiotics is to cease. It is also important to know the stages of healing, what the tissue looks like at each stage, and how dressings affect wounds and their appearance. This will be looked at in Section 5.4.

**Self-assessment**      10 MINUTES

1. How would you define the term colonisation?
2. What does a wound swab identify for you, and why might this be misleading?

3. List five of the criteria which point towards infection in a patient's wound.

## FEEDBACK

You should have said the following.

1. Colonisation is the presence of normal amounts of bacteria on the surface of the wound, which do not interfere with the normal cells.
2. A wound swab identifies the skin bacteria only, which may not be the underlying cause of the infection.
3. You could have given any of the factors listed in Table 5.1, but it is important to remember that usually you would expect to see more than one, but not all, of them.

## 5.4 WOUND ASSESSMENT AND CARE PLANNING

The main purpose for assessing wounds can be summed up as follows:

- to help select the correct dressing for the wound
- to help plan care relating to that wound
- to enable evaluation of treatment measures to take place.

Pressure sores are wounds healing by secondary intention and, as has now been shown, many different factors contribute to their occurrence and whether they heal or not. Assessment of the wound needs to be thorough so that the correct dressing can be chosen to maximise wound healing, and re-assessment should be carried out to evaluate the effectiveness of the chosen dressing.

### Wound assessment

Pressure sore grading systems have already been mentioned, and while some contain subsections which do in fact relate to describing the type of wound, others do not. Even those that do give sub-categories do not always cover every eventuality, which is why it may be best to use a pressure sore grading system and a wound assessment together. While grading systems cover depths of wound, other factors which need to be considered in the process of assessment include the following.

**Site.** Where the wound is may be critical to the choice of dressing. For example, if it is on a heel, a dressing is needed which will conform to the contours; if it is on the sacrum, the dressing may be liable to contamination from faecal or urinary incontinence.

**Colour.** This may indicate infection, that wound healing is progressing well, or that there is slough or necrotic tissue which needs removing for healing to occur.

**Exudate.** The type of exudate provides information about the wound. For example pus would indicate infection; clear serous fluid is often produced when wounds are granulating. Also the amount of exudate is important, as it may be causing a major problem to the staff and patient. Measuring exudate in the ordinary work situation is not easy, and it is sometimes easier to indicate the frequency of dressing changes which will show if there is a problem.

**Odour.** A malodorous wound can have major implications for a patient and his/her family, and can lead to depression and social isolation (van Toller 1994); it is also usually indicative of a problem with the wound which will delay healing, such as the presence of slough or infection.

**Size.** Some measure of size is essential to see whether wounds are improving or not. Several ways exist of measuring wounds, and while some of them such as wound grids have been criticised as not being totally accurate, it is impractical to resort to high technology in many cases, and not necessary. One of the easiest to use is the grid, several of which are now available from commercial companies. An example is shown in Figure 5.1. These can also be placed in the patient's notes, as a permanent record. Additionally, a follow-up grid can be compared to the previous one by counting the number of squares to see if the wound has decreased in size. The squares can also be coloured in to indicate different tissue types in the wound. Photographs are also useful, provided that an indication of size is given. Some cameras now have grids which fit over them and appear on the photograph with the wound to give the size in squares, like the wound grids. Photographs have the added advantage of showing the wound appearance as well.

Patient's Name:                    Date:

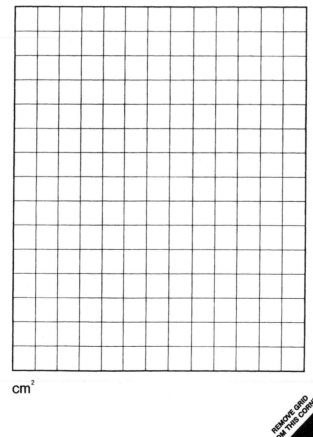

cm$^2$

1. Remove film from card backing using thumb-cut.
2. Place over wound and draw outline on grid using waterproof/indelible pen.
3. Peel apart two films.
4. Tear off along perforation.
5. Retain grid for patient's file.
6. Discard other film.

**Fig. 5.1** Example of a grid for measuring wounds (reproduced by kind permission of Convatec Ltd).

**Depth.** This is more difficult to measure. If there is a cavity with no sinuses, saline can be put into it from a syringe and the depth measured by volume. For example, a wound may take 2 ml this week and 3 ml next week, indicating, provided there has been no change in wound area, that it is getting deeper. This does depend on people filling the cavity to the same depth each time. Another method is to insert a probe gently into a wound or cavity, measuring the depth by how much of it goes in.

More complex systems for measuring area and volume are such things as video image analysis, structured light and laser triangulation, but the majority of pressure sores are unlikely to have these types of measurements done on them. Plassman (1995) provides a useful update, and looks at some of the different ways of measuring wounds, including the advantages and disadvantages of each.

## Activity | 10 MINUTES

Article 11 in the Reader (p. 144) reinforces much of what has already been mentioned in this pack. Look through it again, then list the different methods used to evaluate Mark's wound.

. . . . . . . . . . . . . . . . . . . . . . . . . . . . . . . . .

## FEEDBACK

You should have said that the methods used to evaluate Mark's wound were:

- measurement
- photographs
- the amount of exudate
- stage of healing, granulating tissue.

. . . . . . . . . . . . . . . . . . . . . . . . . . . . . . . . .

## Care planning

This is a method of planning and evaluating patient care following on from total patient assessment. Planning for treatment of pressure sores should be based on wound assessment and knowledge of how wound dressings work. With the possibility of nurse prescribing, which will cover wound dressings, it is essential that nurses are able to devise a care plan which justifies their decision to choose a particular dressing. Nurse prescribing will be looked at in Section 8.2. A typical example of a care plan relating to wound care is shown in Table 5.2.

*Note:* Throughout these sections, dressings will be referred to in their groups, depending on the material they are made of. There are several hydrocolloids and it is likely that you use a specific one in your area, but to avoid bias within this pack, the generic term will be used for the activities that follow. Full lists of products can be obtained from Morgan (1995) and the groups are discussed in Section 5.5.

## Activity | 45 MINUTES

1. Look at the care plan in Table 5.2 and think carefully about it. How useful do you think it is as an initial assessment?
2. Using the care plan in Table 5.3, fill in the last three columns so that it becomes a useful planning tool.
3. In evaluating the effectiveness of the plan, what indicators would you look for that would show that healing was taking place?

. . . . . . . . . . . . . . . . . . . . . . . . . . . . . . . . .

**Table 5.2** Care plan 1: an example of how care plans are often written

| Problem | Aim | Treatment | Evaluation |
|---|---|---|---|
| Sacral sore with some slough | To heal | Hydrocolloid as necessary | |

**Table 5.3** Care plan 2

| Problem | Aim | Treatment | Evaluation |
|---|---|---|---|
| Sacral pressure sore, 2 × 3 cm, with some slough in centre (see graph or photograph) | | | |
| No excess exudate | | | |
| Odour distressing to patient | | | |

## FEEDBACK

1. The site of the sore is given and the fact that there is some slough; what is not included, and should be, is:

   • size of the wound and the sloughy area; there should also be a graph or photograph
   • whether there is any exudate
   • information about odour, which almost definitely will be a problem to a patient with a sloughy wound.

2. Think about this wound—is the aim at this stage to heal? We have already said in Section 5.2 that slough delays wound healing. Is it not therefore your aim to remove the slough? This in fact is what will guide the dressing selection. The stated aim at this stage should be to deslough the wound which will shape your planned care. Additionally, there is no time span given for dressing changes to occur.

3. Evaluation. This column is often left blank because the rest of the care plan has not been filled in such a way as to provide criteria by which evaluation can take place. In this case there was no measurement, so size could not be evaluated; the aim of healing the wound could not be achieved until the wound had been desloughed, so the evaluation of healing would be that none had occurred. Because there was no time schedule for the dressing changes, the effectiveness of the dressing to the wound could not be evaluated. See Table 5.4 for an example of a more meaningful care plan.

   At the end of 2–3 days the dressing would be re-assessed to see whether it was suitable for the wound and the patient. Evaluation could then be weekly and would look at:

   • whether the wound was desloughing
   • whether the dressing was staying in place for 3 days

• whether the patient was finding the odour less troublesome.

Based on this the wound product may or may not remain the same following each evaluation. If the wound was then clean and not smelling it would also be the time to rewrite the care plan and perhaps change the dressing.

This activity covers the main aspects and problems relating to care planning in wound care. However, certain words and phrases frequently crop up which should not be used in the context of care planning because they are meaningless. Examples of these are:

• Large/small—meaning what? They may also mean different things to different people, depending on their previous experience of pressure sores.
• Oozing ++—oozing what, pus, blood, serous fluid? and what is ++?
• Wound is improving—from when? How can you tell if you have not measured and described it?
• Wound looks worse—worse than what and when?

Care planning should be concise, and objective not subjective, particularly when there may have been a complaint about care given and the nursing notes are required to answer the complaint (see Sect. 6.1). It should provide a true picture of the problem, a logical strategy to resolve this, and a treatment plan based on the problem and up-to-date knowledge on which evaluation of care can be based.

Examples of aims for wounds relating to their condition are given in Table 5.5.

You may encounter mixed wounds such as the one in Plate 2 (between pp. 22 and 23) and with these you will have two different aims in the wound healing cycle. You will often have more than one of the factors mentioned, for example a granulating wound can also exude heavily, and all this will affect your choice of wound dressing.

| Table 5.4 Care plan 3 | | | |
|---|---|---|---|
| *Problem* | *Aim* | *Treatment* | *Evaluation* |
| Sacral pressure sore, 2 × 3 cm, with some slough in centre (see graph or photograph) | To deslough | Hydrogel or hydrocolloid Change every 3 days | In 1 week |
| No excess exudate | | | |
| Odour distressing to patient | Control odour | Use carbon dressing | In 2 days |

**Table 5.5** Care plan aims for wounds in relation to their condition

| Condition of wound | Aim of treatment |
|---|---|
| Sloughy | To deslough |
| Necrotic | To debride |
| Infected | To control infection |
| Heavily exuding | Control amount of exudate and reduce dressing changes |
| Granulating | Promote healing (the only time to use this blanket phrase) |
| Malodorous | Control/reduce odour |
| Over-granulation | Reduce granulation |
| Sinus | Prevent healing from top down |

## Activity　　　1½–2 HOURS

Take three patients on your caseload who you see with wounds healing by secondary intention, preferably pressure sores. For each of them, look at the existing care plan and answer the following questions.

1. Have you accurately described the wound?
2. Has this description helped you choose the dressing in use?
3. Can you evaluate the effect of the dressing?

## FEEDBACK

If you can answer 'yes' to all of these, that is very good, but if not do the following.

a. Rewrite the 'Problem' and 'Aim' parts of the care plans, using the list in Table 5.5.
b. Try to get hold of a grid or camera. If you cannot do this, the clear wrapper from a sterile pack can be placed over the wound, enabling you to draw around the wound.
c. In the 'Treatment' column, pencil in the dressing you would choose. Is it any different from the one in use now, and has your assessment changed your mind?
d. Keep hold of these notes as we will use them in the next section when we have looked at wound dressings and you will be asked to fill in the 'Treatment' column properly, together with the 'Evaluation' column, which may or may not indicate that you have increased your knowledge of wound dressings. Has this activity highlighted

any shortfalls in your own care planning. If so make a list in Box 5.1 to help you improve your planning in future.

## Self-assessment　　　20 MINUTES

1. What are the reasons for accurately assessing wounds?
2. Care plans relating to wounds should have four elements. What are they?

## FEEDBACK

1. The reasons for accurately assessing wounds are:

   a. to assist in the correct selection of dressings
   b. to plan the correct care
   c. to enable wound evaluation to take place.

2. All care plans should contain:

   a. concise objective statements of the problems, including a description of the wound and any specific problems being encountered by the patient
   b. the aim, based on the problems
   c. the chosen treatment, based on the problems and up-to-date knowledge of current nursing practice and dressing products
   d. the evaluation, which allows you to check whether the chosen treatment has resolved the problems identified.

**Box 5.1** Steps to improve future care planning

## 5.5 WOUND DRESSINGS

Having looked at how to assess a wound to help select the correct wound dressing, it is important to know how wound dressings work, and what different ones are for. Like pressure-relieving systems, there are many on the market, and more appearing every day. As already mentioned, these modern dressings are perceived by some to be expensive, and indeed they are if incorrectly used, but if they speed up healing and reduce nursing time and patient suffering, it is difficult to see how this argument can be maintained. Having assessed the wound thoroughly so that you know what it is that you want a wound dressing to do, other factors also need to be considered. It is relevant to note here that medical staff are responsible for prescribing dressings, but the reality is that they often depend on the nursing staff advising them on this, especially as they have not always seen the wound recently.

### Ideal environment

In the local environment at the wound face, the following are all factors which will aid healing.

- Moist (not macerated) environment, the advantage of this being that cells can migrate across the moist surface, thus speeding up the healing process. Also a moist environment reduces the pain as the nerve endings are not exposed to the air.
- Free from contamination, which can be chemical or physical, for example anything which sheds fibres into the wound, such as cotton wool or gauze, or inappropriate use of some solutions which can damage healing tissue. This will be looked at under dressing types. Contamination would also include the presence of slough or necrotic tissue on the wound.
- Free from infection.
- Maintained at body temperature.
- Disturbed as little as possible.

Factors to consider when choosing a wound dressing are:

- cost-effectiveness, which is different from basic cost, as will be shown later
- acceptability to patient—a dressing is of no use if the patient removes it at the first opportunity
- ease of application and removal
- availability for use—Section 5.6 looks at some of the problems faced by community staff in relation to this
- valid evidence that the dressing will do what you are expecting it to do for individual wound types.

**Activity**　　　　10 MINUTES

Look again at Article 11 in the Reader (p. 144) and then list the factors that were taken into account when the dressing choice was made for Mark's wound.

**FEEDBACK**

You should have noted that staff took into account all of the following:

- grading and measurement of the wound
- identification of the amount of exudate as a problem, and then use of research articles to help select an effective dressing
- assessment of Mark's physiological and pathological state.

Note that they also started to use an air-fluidised bed to help them manage the wound.

### Types of wound dressings

A brief summary of wound dressings is given below, with one or two examples of each, but by no means all. Suggestions for further reading are given at the end of this section.

#### *Primary dressings*

These are dressings that can go next to the wound surface.

**Semipermeable.** This category used to include only the film dressings, but there are now new ones on the market with some absorbency—examples include Spyrosorb and Tielle. They maintain a moist wound environment, and protect from bacterial invasion.

**Hydrocolloids.** These consist of a matrix which forms a gel on wound contact, and an outer waterproof and protective layer. They come in varying thicknesses, and some have adhesive borders, or bevelled edges to help with adhesion. They can be left in situ for up to 1 week. Examples are Tegaderm, Granuflex and Comfeel.

**Foams.** There are three types: Silastic foam (now known as Cavicare) which is poured into a cavity wound and then sets to the shape of the wound; Lyofoam, a double layer polyurethane dressing which now comes in extra and normal absorbencies; and Allevyn which is both hydrocellular and hydrophilic, increasing its absorbency. It comes in flat sheets, and shapes to fit cavity wounds.

**Hydrogels.** These are hydrophilic gels which absorb fluid from the wound site, and provide an excellent environment for autolysis to occur. There are two types: gels from a tube or sachet which are squeezed on to the wound, such as Intrasite; and flat sheets such as Geliperm or Spenco second skin. These dressings are very versatile, and also very kind to the patient, soothing the wound, and being easy to remove. The gel types will always require a secondary dressing.

**Alginates.** These are made from seaweed. On contact with moisture, the fibres of these dressings start to form a gel, which then maintains the moist environment necessary for wound healing. These are also easy to remove on dressing change. Because of differences in the seaweeds used to make alginates, some form a softer gel in a shorter time, whereas others take longer to form a firmer gel. These products should not be used on dry wounds and need a secondary dressing. Two well-known brands in this country are Sorbsan and Kaltostat and both include an extra-absorbent dressing and a ribbon for packing cavities. Some other alginates are beginning to appear on the market. Kaltosat dressings are also registered as haemostats, that is, they stop bleeding.

**Xerogels.** These are hydrophilic beads and powders such as Debrisan and Iodoflex which also contains iodine.

**Enzymes.** Products such as Varidase are expensive and require a minimum of daily dressing changes, but can be useful in speeding up the debriding process. They must be able to access the wound, so wounds covered with thick necrotic tissue should be scored, or the Varidase injected underneath. This should only be done by a skilled practitioner.

**Low-adherent dressings.** These often stick to the wound, and fail to maintain the ideal healing environment, but improvements have been made recently (e.g. silicone NA and Mepitel) and these can have a particular use where the surrounding skin is fragile.

**Tulle gras.** This fails to meet the criteria for an ideal wound dressing.

**Iodine viscose.** Dressings such as Inadine can be used with systemic antibiotics to treat bacterial infections.

**Gauze.** There can be no justification for using gauze next to wounds in this day and age and with all the modern alternatives. It sheds fibres into the wound, is painful for the patient on dressing changes, and does not maintain the ideal wound-healing environment. It is usually used to apply other substances to the wound such as saline, Eusol and proflavine. These dressings invariably dry out before they are changed, causing pain and damage to the wound bed on removal. There has been much debate on the use of the last two products, particularly Eusol, and, while it may have a very limited place as a short sharp desloughing agent, its use on granulating tissue is not recommended (Farrow & Toth 1990). Aside from the usual debate on the effect these agents have on tissue, it is difficult to see how anyone can continue to use them when the fact is taken into account that they need changing at least daily, and cause unnecessary pain to patients undergoing treatment with them.

**Other dressings.** Some dressings are combined with carbon for controlling odour, examples being Kaltocarb and Actisorb. There are also secondary dressings such as Denidor, which also do this. As community nurses do not have access to any carbon dressings, they may need to resort to alternative odour control methods, such as lavender oil on external dressings, or Nilodor, a product used in stoma care, unless they wish to purchase carbon dressings out of local budgets.

With all the dressings it is essential that users are aware of the makers' recommendations regarding use, and any research which may have been done indicating effectiveness or problems; for example some are not recommended for infected wounds, and dressings containing iodine can cause sensitivities. It is also essential that you know how to apply them, as it has been known for dressings to be applied upside down, an expensive misuse of products.

Another problem is that nursing staff tend to make wound dressing choices based on personal preference, and in the author's experience do not always adhere to the care plan, resulting in changes of dressings in use with each change of nurse. In this age of the named nurse or team nursing this should not occur, as the person who has assessed the wound and planned the care should expect the plan to be followed. The patient should also be involved in this process. Any disagreements on this should be discussed at staff meetings or case conferences. It does the morale of patients no good to see their dressings changed with each nurse, particularly if they have been involved in the discussions relating to their care. Table 5.6 shows the aims of wound care, for example to debride, and suggestions for effective groups of dressings to achieve each aim. There is no hard and fast rule, and you need to consider all the other options mentioned. The list may not be exhaustive, but contains the dressings most commonly available.

**Table 5.6** Aims of wound care and suggested options

| Aim | Suggested option |
| --- | --- |
| To debride | Hydrogel<br>Hydrocolloid<br>Semipermeable |
| To deslough | Hydrogel<br>Hydrocolloid<br>Xerogel |
| To control exudate: | |
| low–medium | Foam<br>Hydrocolloid<br>Alginate<br>New semipermeable |
| medium–high | Extra-absorbent foam<br>Extra-absorbent alginate<br>Hydrocellular foam |
| To control odour | Alginate and carbon dressing*<br>Foam and carbon dressing* |
| Cavity dressing | Pouring foam*<br>Alginate ribbon*<br>Foam fillers* |
| To promote healing | Lyofoam<br>Hydrocolloid<br>Hydrogel<br>New semipermeable |
| For over-granulation | Lyofoam |

* Not available on FP10.

## Activity

**2 HOURS**

1. Look back to the activity you started in Section 5.4 (p. 77) in which you prepared a care plan for three of your patients, and where you have written down any problems related to the wound and the aim of care for that wound. You will also have pencilled in a suitable dressing. Think again of the dressings available to you in your care setting, and with your new knowledge write down the dressing you would choose for this wound, and when you will evaluate its effectiveness.
2. To complete this activity, carry out the evaluation at the time specified, which should not be further away than 2 weeks, and note any differences in carrying out this process from the way in which you did it previously.

## FEEDBACK

1. In reviewing your original care plan did you notice any change in (a) the dressing you had been using, (b) the dressing you pencilled in and (c) your final dressing choice? Was your final choice of dressing based on logical decision making or random choice? Any choice you make will depend on your patients and their wounds. For example if your aim is to control the high amount of exudate, and reduce dressing changes from twice daily, your choice of dressings could be:

 • for a cavity wound, hydrocellular cavity fillers or alginate ribbon covered by hydrocellular foam. Flat dressing only in the community.
 • for a flat wound, extra-absorbent foam or alginate, or hydrocellular foam.

 You will probably have also named the brand that you use, such as Sorbsan or Kaltostat for the alginates. Choice in the community is restricted.

2. When evaluating the wound:

 • Did you find it easier to evaluate your wound care against the aims you had set yourself?
 • Did you feel that your choice of wound product was more appropriate?
 • Did you achieve your aim?
 • Were you able to reduce the number of times you had to do the dressing?
 • Did the patient notice any improvements, for example less pain/odour etc.?

 Your evaluation may result in an update of your care plan, perhaps necessitating a change of wound dressing, or you may be able to stay with the present plan, but possibly reduce the number of dressing changes.

## Additional factors

There are several other factors which need to be considered in relation to dressings, and these include:

 • allergies
 • cost
 • community constraints
 • education.

### Allergies

These are uncommon with modern products, although they do occasionally occur. More frequently, what is described as an allergy is actually the result of an incorrect choice of wound dressing, resulting in inadequate uptake of exudate, which then lies on the surface next to the wound. Exudate, being acid, attacks the skin causing excoriation, which is then classified as an allergy to the wound dressing. More commonly, some of the tapes used to secure a dressing can cause a skin reaction, or damage and tearing where skin is fragile. There may also be a fungal skin infection and, if this is suspected, treatment should be given. Faecal or urinary incontinence may also cause skin problems. It is important to find out the cause of skin problems, and not simply label them as dressing allergies.

## Cost

The cost of a dressing is its base cost, and there is no doubt that modern wound dressings cost more than gauze, non-adherent dressings, surgical pads, etc. However, cost-effectiveness should be based on:

- the frequency of dressing changes (includes nurse time, dressing packs used, etc.)
- rate of healing—if a wound heals in a shorter period of time, the cost of care is lower
- increased patient comfort and acceptability.

Expensive use of wound dressings almost always occurs because the care planning process has not been properly done to facilitate correct dressing choice, or because the nurse is not aware of other options which may be more suitable. Examples would include:

- Using a hydrocolloid on a site where faecal or urinary contamination occurs frequently, necessitating one or more daily dressing changes.
- Continuing to use a normal absorbency product where an extra-absorbent one would be more suitable.
- Constant change of dressing types by individual staff, regardless of care plans. To overcome this, some areas introduce wound formularies. These give a limited number of dressing choices for a type of wound; for example, necrotic wounds —debride with a hydrocolloid or enzyme. Any other dressing choice will not be sanctioned or dispensed without specific reasons. Formularies need to be compiled by a small group of users, such as pharmacists, nurses and medical staff, and then introduced to all users who should have a copy for reference. They should also be suitable for use across care boundaries. Dressing costs may well be reduced by more appropriate use and cutting out the element of dressing choice based on personal preference only. Formularies need to be evaluated annually, and user-comments and recent research considered, as changes may need to be made to update them. Blaber (1993) describes how a wound formulary was implemented in a health district.
- Community constraints (see Sect. 5.6).
- Education—this needs to be constant and ongoing, based on how, when and where to use

wound products, and again this is where a link nurse can have a useful role as the identified person to be educated, and keep up to date with research, so that he/she can pass the knowledge on to other members of staff.

Self-assessment          30 MINUTES

1. List five conditions that a dressing should create at the wound site in order to encourage wound healing.

2. Which other four factors must be considered when choosing a dressing?

3. Name two products which could be used for each of the following situations:

   a. to control medium to high amounts of exudate
   b. to debride a wound by autolysis
   c. to fill a cavity wound.

4. What aspects need to be considered when looking at whether or not a dressing is cost effective?

## FEEDBACK

1. The conditions at the wound site which encourage wound healing are:

   - moisture at the wound surface
   - freedom from contamination
   - freedom from infection
   - maintenance at body temperature
   - as little disturbance as possible.

2. Other factors include:

   - cost-effectiveness
   - acceptability to patient
   - ease of application and removal
   - availability
   - proven evidence of performance.

3. a. Products which could be used to control medium to high exudate are:

   - extra-absorbent alginate
   - hydrocellular foam
   - extra-absorbent foam.

   b. Products which could be used for autolysis are:

   - hydrocolloid
   - hydrogel
   - semipermeable dressing.

c. Products which could be used to fill a cavity are:

- a cavity foam filler
- alginate packing
- paste
- hydrogel.

4. Cost-effectiveness is affected by the number of dressing changes required, the rate of healing and patient comfort and acceptability.

●●●●●●●●●●●●●●●●●●●●●●●●●●●●●●●●●●●

Having answered these questions you should now feel that you have a better knowledge base of dressings, although it must be stressed that this is only a brief overview, and further reading of the references is recommended along with specialist journals such as the *Journal of Wound Care* to obtain a greater depth of knowledge. In addition, this has been written with only pressure sores in mind, and not the other types of wounds that occur.

## 5.6 COMMUNITY CONSTRAINTS

The previous two subsections have shown that choosing a dressing relates to several factors, particularly wound assessment, but also other aspects. There is, however, one further consideration for those staff working in the community setting and that is the fact that their dressing choice can only be based on what is available on the drug tariff, regardless of whether or not they are the most appropriate products to use. In future, GPs as purchasers may be able to overcome this, as practices with lists of 3000–5000 patients will be given limited purchasing power, including budgets for drugs and dressings (Young 1995).

### The drug tariff

This is an attempt by the Government to provide value for money by providing GPs with a range of dressings for their patients, while keeping costs down by not supplying the same range of products that are available to the acute sector. To get a product included on the drug tariff, its safety, quality and efficacy have to be proved (Young 1994). Despite the fact that many dressings meet these criteria, they are still not included on the tariff, a decision made by civil servants at the Department of Health. That this has always been a contentious issue for those working in the community is well known, and there have been some improvements recently, with the apparent acceptance that there are wounds in the community measuring more than 10 cm × 10 cm, and consequential inclusion of the larger dressing sizes

in the foam and hydrocolloid range. Additionally, some of the new semipermeable products have recently come on to the tariff. However, the main exclusions are:

- products to cope with heavily exuding wounds
- cavity dressings
- dressings to cope with malodorous wounds.

It is exactly these wounds and these types of problems which can cause most distress to patients and their carers.

Section 1.2 discussed the demographic changes that are leading to the potential for more patients to develop pressure sores in their own homes, and the whole change in health care settings, with the shift to primary care, means that many patients are discharged with wounds and pressure sores, where previously they would have been kept in hospital, at least until healing was well underway. Also needing to be taken into account are leg ulcers, which are almost exclusively cared for in the community setting (see Moffat & Harper 1997 for further reading on this subject). An additional problem is that, despite the fact that nurses now complete some of their training in the community, once they revert to the acute sector, they seem unaware of the problems experienced by district nurses and the private sector in acquiring dressings. This is a double problem, highlighting a lack of education and communication.

**Activity**   20 MINUTES

Article 13 in the Reader (p. 150) gives a good overview of some of the problems relating to community wound care and why products are excluded from the drug tariff.

1. Read the article then list the main problems which it identifies relating to the drug tariff.
2. What, according to the article, is the main outcome of the system for patients?

●●●●●●●●●●●●●●●●●●●●●●●●●●●●●●●●

## FEEDBACK

1. You should have identified the following problems:

- financial problems, perceived as overspending by GP fundholders, and the reluctance of hospitals to fund community dressings for a patient since the advent of trusts
- lack of knowledge by hospital staff of the constraints on wound care experienced in the community

- lack of hospital and community communication, and specifically when devising wound formularies.

2. The article identified that as a result of the drug tariff a two-tier system of patient care is being practised in relation to wound care, with community patients as the losers.

## Financial problems

This comes back to the difference discussed in Section 5.5 between base cost and cost-effectiveness. A dressing which improves the healing of a wound, reduces district nurse visits and helps patients to cope with their wounds, may have a base cost higher than an alternative, but is more cost effective. Note the effect on the patient, Mrs Smith, quoted in Reader Article 10 (p. 142), and obviously the deteriorating progress of this wound would have entailed more district nurse time. The article also made the point that the dressings most suited to improving the patient's quality of life were often not available in the community, but had to be specially supplied by the research nurse. With the Patients' Charter, and increasing patient knowledge, it is difficult to see how this situation can continue.

## Lack of knowledge

This comes back to education. Young (1994) discovered that one reason the DoH were reluctant to put more dressings on the drug tariff was because of surveys showing variable knowledge among district nurses on the use of dressings. Recommendations were made to include wound management courses for pre- and post-registration nurses. As there have been similar surveys relating to hospital staff (O'Connor 1993), the argument seems somewhat flawed and it is also debatable whether this is a valid reason for denying patients the most effective care for their wounds. Nowadays there are many study days on wound care, all well attended. The link nurse would also help to solve the problem of lack of knowledge.

## Communication

The hospital/community divide can be breached. Article 12 in the Reader (p. 147) notes how ward staff were supplied with an up-to-date list of the products available on the drug tariff, and the same approach has been taken using the discharge flow chart shown in Section 4 (Fig. 4.1, p. 61). Again the link nurses can be encouraged to take the lead in this, and joint meetings between community and hospital staff are

useful in removing barriers. District nurses can be encouraged to visit patients with large wounds before they are discharged, if the geographical proximity allows, and certainly community staff should have adequate warning of the discharge of these types of patients, and be asked to attend any discharge case conferences.

**Activity**      10 MINUTES

### *Hospital staff*

Think of the last patient you discharged with a grade 3 or over pressure sore, or if this does not apply, any other type of wound. Now answer the following questions.

1. Were the dressings in use available to the community staff?
2. Were community staff involved in or notified of the discharge as soon as you knew the patient was going to be discharged?

### *Community staff*

1. Was the last patient discharged into your care with a grade 3 or over pressure sore on dressings that were available to you on FP10?
2. Were you involved in/notified of the discharge as soon as planning began?

### *All staff*

Regardless of the answers given above, but particularly if they indicate communication gaps, how do you think things could be improved in your area?

## FEEDBACK

The answers relating to the individual patients will vary, but even if things went well this time, it is likely that you can think of occasions when problems have arisen.

You may feel that your area would benefit from:

- a discharge chart showing dressings available on the drug tariff
- a wound formulary compiled between community and acute staff
- an education programme or joint meetings with both sets of staff.

Perhaps you see some way of moving this forward.

Young (1994) sees the way forward as improving communication and education, but she also feels that the size of the problem needs defining for the DoH to be encouraged to act. Some quality of life studies relating to patients, in particular in relation to some of the issues we have already discussed in other sections, may prove useful. Remember John in Reader Article 6 (p. 124) and how the dressing improved his quality of life, and the reference in Section 5.4 to how odour can affect a patient's life. If community care is the goal for the majority of patients, then it is time they had access to the same resources as hospital patients.

## SUMMARY

In this section you have learned:

- the process of wound healing
- as a nurse caring for patients with wounds, it is essential to have a basic knowledge of wound healing and factors which assist and delay the process
- accurate wound assessment and care planning are of great importance in wound care
- the choice of dressing for a wound depends on many factors, including appropriateness to the local environment, cost-effectiveness, acceptability to the patient and availability
- a number of constraints exist which affect wound care in the community.

REFERENCES

Bennett G, Moody M 1995 Wound care for health professionals. Chapman & Hall, London
Blaber C 1993 Centred on excellence. Journal of Wound Care Nursing, Nursing Times 89(49): 1–4
Cox D 1993 Growth factors in wound healing. Journal of Wound Care 2(6): 339–342
Cutting K, Harding K 1994 Criteria for identifying wound infection. Journal of Wound Care 3(4): 198–201
Dealey C 1994a The care of wounds. Blackwell Scientific Publications, London
Dealey C 1994b A prevention and management aid: evaluation of the Nimbus II Mattress. Professional Nurse 9(12): 798–804
Farrow S, Toth B 1990 The place of Eusol in wound management. Health Care Evaluation Unit, Bristol
James J 1995 Low power laser therapy. Journal of Community Nursing (March): 20–26
Lowthian P 1995 Pegasus Airwave and Biwave Plus. British Journal of Nursing 4(17): 1020–1024
Morgan D 1995 Formulary of wound care products, 5th edn. Media Medica Publications, Chichester
O'Connor H 1993 Bridging the gap. Journal of Wound Care 5(4): 1–4
Perry C 1996 Methicillin-resistant *Staphylococcus aureus*. Journal of Wound Care 5(1): 31–34
Plassman R 1995 Measuring wounds. Journal of Wound Care 4(6): 269–272
Ryan D 1990 The fluidised bed: basic principles, bacteriology and wound care. Intensive Care World 7(2): 92–96
Smith & Nephew and RCN 1991 Wound management education system, module 3. Smith & Nephew, Hull
Van Toller S 1994 Invisible wounds: the effects of skin ulcer malodours. Journal of Wound Care 3(2): 103–105
Young L 1995 GP fund holders must listen to us. Community Nurse (February): 9
Young T 1994 Wound management: the hospital community divide. British Journal of Nursing 4(14): 702–706

FURTHER READING

Flanagan M 1997 Wound management. (Access to Clinical Education Series) Churchill Livingstone, Edinburgh
Moffatt C, Harper P 1997 Leg ulcers. (Access to Clinical Education Series) Churchill Livingstone, Edinburgh
Morgan D A 1994 Formulary of wound management, 6th edn. Euromed Communications, Haslemere
Thomas S (ed) 1994 Handbook of wound dressings. Journal of Wound Care, London

# 6 Specific issues

This section looks at issues that, so far, have been touched on in the text but not discussed in detail. These are ethics, aspects of law, business planning and changing practice. Ethics affect all nurses and if progress is to be made, nurses need to look at changing practice. Business planning is increasingly important in these times of limited resources to help obtain what is needed for your area.

## LEARNING OUTCOMES

At the end of this section you will be able to:

- identify ethical dilemmas which can arise in pressure sore management and the legal issues raised
- recognise problems relating to resources and how to try to overcome them
- identify obstacles which may face nurses trying to change existing practice.

## 6.1 ETHICS AND LAW

In health care, ethical issues relate not just to life and death issues but often to more mundane, but nevertheless difficult, patient care problems. Two ethical views are the deontological and the teleological, which offer two extremes. Teleologists are those who believe in an action or in achieving goals, regardless of the cost to individuals. Deontologists believe in the rights of the person regardless of the consequences. To take either of these extremes in health care does not address the many complex issues concerned, not least the rights and responsibilities of the patients and the nurses. Tschudin (1994) puts forward another theory of response ethics, based on work by Niebuhr (1963), in which four main areas should be taken into account in any decisions made in ethical dilemmas. These are:

- relationships
- rights and responsibilities
- personal and professional issues
- needs of people and the system.

## Relationships

Relationships have a profound effect on patients, in particular their relationship with the health care worker, although all other relationships need to be taken into account. Health care decisions made by patients are based on the patients' level of autonomy which is described by Tingle (1988) as being in a state of self-control and self-direction. Many ill patients are in neither state, because of loss of independence as a result of their illness, their limited knowledge in relation to their illness and treatment, and the imbalance of power which exists between the health care worker and the patient as a result of this (Carpenter 1992).

A key to making autonomous decisions is that the person involved has all the facts and understands them.

**Activity**      10 MINUTES

Using your own experience, write down three ways in which you can help a patient to make informed decisions.

## FEEDBACK

To help a patient make informed decisions, you could have suggested:

- making sure that the patient has received a full explanation in non-medical jargon of what is wrong with him/her and the consequences of not undertaking the chosen treatment together with an explanation of any alternative treatment methods available
- providing any available written information on the subject, such as a patient information leaflet
- ensuring that the patient has been given the time and opportunity to ask questions, and does not feel too intimidated by surroundings or personnel to do so.

Being able to do any of these will depend to some extent on the relationship between health care workers and patients. An additional dilemma for nurses can often be that if patients make decisions with which other medical staff do not agree, it is often the nurse to whom the patients look to support them in their decisions. If as a result of patients' choices a pressure sore develops, who is then responsible?

**Activity** 10 MINUTES

Think of a patient in your care who has refused to comply with nursing care and then look at the three points mentioned above. Can you honestly say that the patient made a fully informed decision? If not, give any reasons why you felt the patient was not given all the information and the chance to question staff.

## FEEDBACK

This will depend on your own area, but it is likely that at least one of the options did not exist or was not used, common reasons given being:

- lack of time on the part of the nursing staff
- lack of knowledge by the nurses
- feeling by medical and nursing staff that 'we know best', particularly in relation to the amount of information given to the patient
- lack of information booklets, maybe in general or maybe just in your area.

## Rights and responsibilities

These relate to both the patient and the nurse. The Patients' Charter (DoH 1995) has reinforced patients' rights, and states that the patient has the right 'to have any proposed treatment, including any risks involved in that treatment and any alternatives clearly explained to you before you decide whether to agree to it.' This, however, totally ignores the patients' responsibilities which are inevitably intertwined with rights. Dimond (1993) in a very useful book summarises patients' rights, but also points out that patients have a responsibility to 'carry out instructions on treatment and care responsibly and carefully, or inform staff if this has not been done.'

To confuse the issue, nurses too have rights and responsibilities, tied in with their professional codes of conduct. Even here all is not clear, because Clause 1 of the professional code (UKCC 1992) expects nurses to always safeguard patients, while Clause 5 expects them to foster independence and involvement of

patients in care planning. As will be shown, the two do not always go together.

Legally all professionals owe a duty of care to their patients. Patients can sue for development of a pressure sore if they can prove that the nursing care has broken down to the extent that foreseeable damage occurs to the patient. However, staff can refute this accusation if they can prove contributory negligence by the patient in refusing to cooperate or accept treatment. This defence will only succeed if it can be proved that the patient was aware of the consequences of any decisions he or she may have made regarding non-compliance with treatment. It will also depend on how well the nursing staff documented all the factors leading up to the incident.

## Personal and professional issues

These depend on how people interpret and use charters and codes such as the two mentioned previously. They will be affected by social factors and the care setting where the patient is being looked after. Personal beliefs by staff or patients may arise here for consideration, an example in general terms being nurses who do not agree with abortion, or a Jehovah's Witness refusing to have a blood transfusion.

## Needs of people and the system

Much of this section ties in with availability of resources and how they are allocated, which is looked at in Section 6.2. But it also relates to whose needs take priority, the people or the system, as very often they conflict. Also, who decides a person's need? Do the health care workers, because they believe they know what is best for patients, or do they really consider or indeed know what the patient needs or wants?

**Activity** 15 MINUTES

Look again at Article 9 in the Reader (p. 140)—Baroness Masham is an example of a patient well aware of her own problems and what is needed to avoid pressure sores. List three factors which contributed to poor care following her return from Mauritius and subsequent hospitalisation.

## FEEDBACK

You should have identified the following factors.

- The GP's lack of understanding of the importance of anaemia in this patient —remember anaemia

is one of the predisposing conditions for
pressure sores.
- The lack of equipment to meet her needs when
  in hospital.
- The lack of understanding of the wound healing
  process and how long it can take in wounds
  healing by secondary intention.

· · · · · · · · · · · · · · · · · · · · · · · · · · · ·

A common scenario in health care is the patient who
is labelled difficult or uncooperative because he or
she fails to do what the health care workers wish.
How often do we look beyond the conflict to find
out the reasons why?

Tschudin (1994) identifies three key questions
which need to be asked by staff when solving ethical
dilemmas, and these are:

- What is happening?
- What is the meaning of it?
- What is the fitting answer? This means the
  answer most suitable to the problem at the time,
  given all the facts.

The answers to the last two questions will depend
on how the nurse interprets Question 1 in the context
of the four ethical areas mentioned (relationships,
rights and responsibilities, personal and professional
issues, and needs of people and the system). The
issue being looked at is refusal of a patient to follow
a planned care intervention, i.e. a patient at risk
of developing pressure sores failing to comply with
suggested prevention strategies, or a patient with
sores failing to comply with relevant treatment.

## Activity                         1–1½ HOURS

1. Box 6.1 presents a true scenario of a patient
   refusing to use pressure-relieving equipment.
   When you have read this:

   a. Answer Tschudin's three key questions:
      —What is happening?
      —What is the meaning of it?
      —What is the fitting answer?
      considering all the factors mentioned.

   b. How do your conclusions compare with the
      action taken by staff?

   c. Would you support the patient's decision?
      Does any conflict arise with the professional
      code of conduct?

2. Think of a patient in your own area who has
   failed to comply with planned care, preferably in
   relation to pressure sore prevention. It could be

---

### Box 6.1 Mrs M

Mrs M was a paraplegic lady in her 60s with
congestive cardiac failure which was deteriorating,
causing discomfort, reduced quality of life and
making more work for her husband who cared for
her. It was also increasing her risk of pressure sore
development because of the further reduction in
mobility and ill health. Despite the district nurse's
efforts, Mrs M was refusing to be nursed on more
sophisticated pressure-relieving equipment. She had
previously had pressure sores, and was therefore
aware of the consequences of one. The district
nurse called in the nurse specialist for back-up,
although she actually accepted the patient's
decision, but wanted to cover herself. The patient
was given a leaflet on pressure sore prevention and
the problems were discussed with her, including the
fact that she may need to be admitted to hospital
should a pressure sore develop. She was persuaded
to try an electric mattress for one night, but then
maintained her previous stance. 3 months later
she was admitted to hospital with extensive
pressure damage. Medical staff began treatment
but within 2 weeks the patient and her husband
discharged her against medical advice to a nursing
home, where she soon died, the pressure sore
having contributed to her death.

---

related to equipment, not eating, continuing to sit
out of bed, not moving or any other intervention.
Answer the same three questions and see
whether it changes your outlook on the problem.
Also ask whether you have honestly given the
patient all the information on which to base
his/her choice.

· · · · · · · · · · · · · · · · · · · · · · · · · · · ·

## FEEDBACK

1. *What is happening?* The patient is refusing to
   accept measures which will assist her carers and
   prevent or delay the onset of pressure sores.

   *What is the meaning of this?* With all the
   information available, the following was the
   interpretation given to the situation. The patient
   was fully aware of what she was doing, she had
   been given information by the staff, and she also
   knew from first hand that pressure sores cause
   major problems. She had not enjoyed a high
   quality of life and that was now further reduced;
   she may also have felt guilt at the extra workload
   on her husband. Her congestive cardiac failure
   left her feeling weak and depressed a lot of the
   time. She was not interested in any interventions
   which might prolong her life. This was supported

by her decision to leave hospital when aggressive treatments were started.

*What is the fitting answer?* There can be no right or wrong here, precisely because it is an ethical dilemma. The specialist nurse was called in and fully supported the district nurse who in turn felt that the patient had made a decision based on all the facts of what was best for her. She was tired of living and wanted no more interventions in her life.

It is interesting to note that when the patient was admitted to hospital the reactions from the staff were:

• Recriminations against the district nurse for allowing the patient to get in such a state. How many times do we make judgements like this between care settings without knowing the full story?
• Disbelief, when she and her husband decided on self-discharge, and continual efforts to get the patient to change her mind, instead of support for a difficult decision.

The district nurse had continued to nurse the patient at home until it was no longer possible and had respected her independence and involvement in her care, even if it was not with the outcomes she might have hoped for. This of course relates to the code of conduct, but could be seen as conflicting with Clause 1 as the patient's well-being in the medical sense had been compromised, but not in the personal and psychological sense.

2. Your own case will depend on the patient and all the facts relating to the case, but may well have caused you to re-examine how you think about and judge patients. It is often easier for community and nursing home staff to make judgements based on the whole picture, as they care for patients for longer periods and, in the case of district nurses, in their own homes. Ironically, this can also make any ethical decisions harder. Did you think your patient fully understood the consequences of his/her action, and why you were asking him/her to comply with that particular aspect of care? Was the patient seriously ill or feeling helpless in the health care setting so that pressure sore prevention measures just seemed another intrusion?

## Record keeping

This is extremely important in relation to legal issues which may arise. Young & Tingle (1995) point out that inadequate records may result in damages being awarded against the nurse or employing authority. They list essential principles of record keeping as:

• Contemporary: completed as near as possible to the time of the care or incident.
• Comprehensive: ensure that the precise response to care is reported as well as the care given. Particularly record any unusual occurrences or observations and any omissions.
• Factual: assumptions must be avoided and opinion clearly stated as such.
• Suitably frequent: frequency depends on the particular circumstances, e.g. every few hours in a critical care environment and weekly in a more stable care setting. Review dates should be set and adhered to.
• Signed and dated: initials are unacceptable.
• Legible: abbreviations can only be included if very common and well known.
• Free of errors: if errors are made, the mistake should be crossed through and the amendment made; both must be signed.
• Permanent: pencil must not be used.

Nurses must learn to document all decisions and the reasons why they were made. If a case ever does come to court it is often many months or even years after the patient was in care, and it is unrealistic to expect the nursing staff to remember what mattress the patient was on or what the patient's risk assessment score was. Additionally, even if there is a complaint, dealing with it to everyone's satisfaction will depend on being able to tell people exactly what happened, when and why. It is also essential to record if a patient refuses to cooperate in planned care as has already been shown. Care plans relating to pressure sore prevention should show:

• risk assessment score and time carried out
• evidence of reassessment as necessary or laid down by local policies
• equipment chosen and when patient started to use it
• a note if patient refused to use it, including details of any explanations or teaching done by staff to try to explain treatment objectives to patient
• if and when equipment was changed or discontinued
• a note of the first time any sign of pressure damage was observed
• any other preventative strategies employed
• notes of any teaching done to carers in relation to prevention.

Saying that something is always done or that you are sure it would have been done, will not stand up in a court of law.

1. What four factors need to be taken into account when considering an ethical dilemma?
2. What is meant by autonomy in the context of patients making decisions about their own health care?
3. Complete the following sentence. When a patient suffers injury as the result of a nurse's action or lack of action, the patient may sue the nurse for failing in her                 . Staff can respond with a claim of                    if the patient, having understood all the consequences, still refuses to comply with treatment or planned care.

## FEEDBACK

You should have said the following.

1. The four factors are:

   • relationships
   • rights and responsibilities
   • personal and professional issues
   • needs of people and systems.

2. Autonomy is defined as a state of self-control and self-being, and patients need to be in possession of all the facts in order to make decisions about their health care.

3. The two missing phrases are: (a) duty of care and (b) contributory negligence.

## 6.2 RESOURCE IMPLICATIONS AND BUSINESS PLANNING

There have been major changes in the management of health care resources in recent years with a new approach which can be summarised in the words of Clarke (1994) as:

• a systematic approach to setting establishments and manpower planning
• assessment prioritisation of the health and nursing needs of the local population
• development of appropriate measures of service outcomes
• detailed establishment design, staff range and skill mix, workload analysis.

In a survey of 64 nursing staff with varying backgrounds by Caldock (1993) over half cited finance and provision of resources as main areas of concern

for implementation of the White Paper on community care (Griffiths 1988). She also points out that it is likely that, with the changes in patient care, fewer resources will be available for more dependent patients in their own homes. Teasdale (1993) recognises that the level of central funding will be a factor in the success of community care, and that it will need a rethink to move the money into areas not previously well funded. A problem is that pressure sores in particular are not seen as glamorous, and are not an area to attract spending. However, the government targets have at least put the problem on everyone's agenda, so now is probably a good time to try to rationalise and seek funding to help solve this problem.

Clarke (1994) identifies two other major factors affecting community nursing as discharge planning and the use of social services home care. She recognises the extra work involved in caring for patients who are often still very dependent, and who have been discharged without proper discharge planning into the community, where the staff are pushed to cope with the patient and the resources are not immediately available. This is particularly true at weekends, when the nursing service is reduced and agencies to set home care in motion are not available, and yet many patients are sent home from hospital on Fridays with no thought to what happens over the weekend. A solution to this is a discharge plan and policy as described in Section 4.5.

The social services home care situation is looked at more fully in Section 8.3 where a case history shows some of the problems that can arise.

Read the case history contained in Box 1 in Article 14 of the Reader (p. 155).

1. What resource problems led to the patient developing a pressure sore?
2. What resource problems existed after the sore occurred?

## FEEDBACK

1. You should have identified the different reasons given for the lack of care by two different managers: first that there were insufficient resources in terms of staff in home care; and second that there were enough staff, but they were not prepared to work in the early morning. This in itself indicates disagreement among the management of the home care workers, but the

fact remains that they were aware of a problem. It also incidentally shows a lack of concern for the patient in human terms and ignorance of factors which can cause pressure sores. It is interesting to note that when a complaint was made, more appropriate care was provided.

2. District nurses had to make more visits to dress the pressure sore. Additionally, although this was not mentioned, the cost of care would have risen with the need for wound dressings. In the author's experience district nurses are not always being involved sufficiently in the assessment and care of patients with medical conditions, or at risk of pressure sore problems, with the result that the first time the district nurse is called in is often to treat a problem rather than prevent one, which can take more time and resources in itself. Solving this involves more education for those working in other care areas and for patients and carers, perhaps by the use of an information leaflet.

## Business planning

People think this is a complex process, but the simpler you keep it the better. There are plenty of books around on the way to do business plans, and that will not be covered in detail here; however, a quick look at the essentials may help to persuade you that it is one way to put your case for more resources. As stated by Clarke (1994), you need to find out the health needs of your population, and we are going to look at this in terms of asking for resources for pressure sore prevention. This then comes back to the size of the problem, which you will need to measure to show that there is a need. This would particularly be in relation to the number of pressure sores which started in your care setting, or the incidence of sores. If you were putting a case for treatment of pressure sores, it would involve the prevalence, or total numbers with sores. When you have the basic information, you can start to make your case.

To do this, you need to know when your business plan has to be ready to go for consideration by the trust management. Speak to your manager and get his or her support to submit a plan, particularly if there are a few of you working together. Do not struggle to manage with inadequate resources; document when problems related to lack of resources arise and show this to your manager, particularly if it compromises patient care. It is essential that nurses become more involved in the business planning process, not least because they are the ones who really know the issues that affect direct patient care. To prepare your case, you should take the following steps.

1. *Analyse the current situation.* You can do this by carrying out a SWOT analysis. SWOT stands for:

   S —strengths, what strengths do you currently have?
   W—weaknesses, what are your current weaknesses?
   O —opportunities, what opportunities do we have for making things better?
   T —threats, what threatens to prevent us from achieving our goals?

2. *State your long- and short-term goals.* A long-term goal might be a comprehensive education programme for patients and carers, which is very much in line with present government thinking on health promotion and home care. Give brief strategies for how you hope to achieve your goals and, most importantly of all, how you intend to show effectiveness and measure quality outcomes of what you are doing.

If you have been realistic and are given money, and are then able to carry out your short-term goals and prove effectiveness, follow this up the next year with a further plan to carry on. Do not be discouraged if you fail to get accepted the first time round; not everyone will succeed, but keep trying.

**Activity**      45 MINUTES

To get you used to thinking in the right way, take an area in your own setting which you would like to see better resourced or improved.

1. Write out your short-term and long-term goals.
2. How would you evaluate the plan? That is, what targets can be set which, when reached, will show that you have achieved your goals?
3. Do a SWOT analysis of the current situation.

Examples of goals might be more equipment at a basic level for your patients, or the ability to provide more education for social services carers or patients and their carers, or the need to rationalise the wound dressings in use by providing a wound formulary.

## FEEDBACK

This will depend on your own area, and what you have chosen as your goals, but taking a request for equipment as an example your answer should look something like the following.

1. Short term goal—to provide enough equipment for the existing patients.

Long term goal—to have enough equipment to be able to allocate resources effectively in the future.
2. Evaluating the short-term goal would mean measuring how many patients should be on equipment at the present time, and are not. Evaluating the plan for the long term goal would require costing out some patient episodes, especially if they developed a pressure sore because of lack of equipment.
3. The strengths, weaknesses, opportunities and threats will depend on your particular circumstances, but the process of identifying them should help you to formulate a plan that builds on the advantages which you already have, takes into account any difficulties and makes the most of the opportunities while avoiding factors which threaten the success of the plan.

Do not make your plan simply a request for lots of expensive equipment; this will be turned down. Be realistic; think of other ways of reducing the pressure sore problem, bearing in mind that this pack has already mentioned that education is the most important factor. Would money to provide patient education booklets help you, along with some lower-scale pressure-relieving/reducing equipment and maybe just a few higher support systems?

This subject is small for a business plan, but it may form part of a bigger whole, or you may simply seek some finance to have posters or educational material published to help with this initiative. It is hoped that this has set you on the road to thinking about how to do a business plan; now all you need to do is think on a bigger scale.

## 6.3 CHANGING PRACTICE

It is unlikely that you have read this pack and not identified at least one area of practice that you would like to see changed. If you hope to achieve this, you need to be aware of some of the problems associated with changing practice. Again, for further detail it is recommended that you read other textbooks, e.g. Carnall (1990), Mabey & Mayon-White (1993), but an overview will be given, looking at the following:

- type of change
- change agent
- reactions to change
- change will involve the whole team.

### Type of change

There are two main types of change, planned and unplanned; this text relates to planned change. To carry out planned change one of the following three strategies can be used:

- empirical rational, which assumes that humans are rational and will follow a change once the benefits are explained
- power coercive, where people with greater power influence those with less power
- normative re-educative, based on assumptions about human motivation.

While power coercive is often the method people try to use, the more appropriate one for health care is likely to be normative re-educative. To achieve this, people need to change their skills, attitudes and values, which then helps to make a new behaviour pattern permanent. Education or re-education, then, is the key to success with this approach. This needs to be tied in with the planned change. Bernhard & Walsh (1981) identify planned change as 'a change with a purpose or goal which is usually the improvement of a system through alteration'. They acknowledge how difficult this can be in the health care setting, which is a bureaucratic system, resistant to change of any sort. Walsh & Ford (1989) give a good insight into some of the problems surrounding change in nursing. Bernhard & Walsh (1981) identify three steps in planned change:

1. unfreezing, which is when people begin to recognise the need for change
2. moving, when the change is implemented, often by a change agent, and by education
3. refreezing, which is when the change has been accepted, and people begin to adopt the changes as normal, and do them all the time.

To instigate change, an action plan is needed, stating what you hope to achieve and the stages you will go through to do this, with dates. An example is given in Box 6.2.

---

**Box 6.2** Action plan to instigate change

**Planned change:** To start using a risk assessment score on all patients

**Plan:**
Discuss with manager: 2.3.96

Form a small group to select most appropriate tool for that area: by 10.3.96

Present to work area and provide opportunities for questions: by 20.3.96

Explain rationale for change and perceived benefits: by 20.3.96

Educate all staff in the use of the tool: complete by 10.4.96

Set a start date and a period for trial of tool: 11.4.96–30.5.96

Evaluate: week of 1.6.96

1. Choose a change that you would like to see in relation to pressure sore prevention or treatment in your area and one which you think you could start to implement.
2. Work out a plan like the one in Box 6.2 in order to bring about the change successfully.

## FEEDBACK

Your answer will depend on the area chosen by you. You should have looked at involving other staff, perhaps by finding out what they feel needs changing so that they are involved in the process. This would fit in with the normative re-educative change theory.

Keep this activity for an exercise later in this section.

## Change agent

The role of the change agent is difficult. In the pressure sore world, this role is often taken on by the clinical nurse specialist, but where there are link nurses they can be expected to perform this in a smaller area, their own work area. Wright (1985) lists 10 qualities (Q) and types of support (S) needed by a change agent as:

- possession of clinical, educational and managerial expertise, appropriate to the setting (Q)
- supportive and approachable managers (S)
- proven written and verbal communication skills (Q)
- physical and psychological stamina (Q)
- philosophy of nursing and objectives (S)
- peer group support (S)
- knowledge of functioning of health care system (Q)
- secretarial support (S)
- positive personal relationships, for support in non-professional life (S)
- commitment to the job (Q).

It is highly unlikely that anyone has all of these, and link nurses at ward level may or may not have supportive managers. Certainly this is a key to successful change in local areas. Staff need to have access to educate and inform other staff whether at small arranged teaching sessions or during ward report, or at staff meetings. Peer group support, such as link nurse meetings, are also useful, and may help people to see that they are not the only ones with problems, while exchange of ideas may help to solve problems in different areas.

## Resistance to change

Change is threatening. Even if the present situation is far from ideal, it represents what is known, and this is one reason why there is always resistance to change. Bernhard & Walsh (1981) identify a resistance/acceptance continuum:

Active resistance—passive resistance—apathy —passive acceptance—active acceptance.

The people who come at either end are in some ways the easiest to deal with as there is no doubt where they stand in the change process. It is the others who can cause problems, particularly the passive resistors, who may not say anything directly to the change agents but will try to undermine their work as soon as they are not around. Many staff will be in the 'apathy' category unless the change is a very emotive one, and these people tend to go for the easiest option, which is not usually to instigate change. It is essential to be aware of all these people and try to have a plan to overcome their resistance. The most effective way to convince people is for them to see results, which may be achieved in wound care, but is not always so obvious in other areas.

Article 15 in the Reader (p. 156) describes how a research project was used to change nursing practice. Read this article and then answer the following questions.

1. How was the study subject chosen?
2. What are the main points that a change agent needs to consider when undertaking change?
3. What did the authors recognise as:
   a. essential in the planning stage for the project to succeed?
   b. responsible for the lack of resistance met during the project?

## FEEDBACK

Your answers should have been as follows.

1. The subject was chosen on the basis of the needs and interests of the staff working on the unit.
2. The main points for a change agent to consider were:
   - An almost universal tendency to seek and maintain the status quo on the part of those whose needs are being met by it.

- Resistance to change increases in proportion to the degree to which it is perceived as a threat.
- Resistance to change increases in direct response to pressure for change.
- Resistance to change decreases when the change is perceived as being reinforced by trusted others, such as high prestige figures, those whose judgement is respected, people of like mind.
- Resistance to change decreases when those involved are able to foresee how they might establish a new equilibrium as good as or better than the old.
- Commitment to change increases when those involved have the opportunity to participate in the decision to make and to implement the change.
- Resistance to change based on fear of the new circumstances is decreased when those involved have the opportunity to experience the new under conditions of minimal threat.
- Temporary alterations in most situations can be brought about by the use of direct pressure, but these changes are accompanied by heightened tension and will yield a highly unstable situation.

3. a. Evaluation of driving and resisting forces before the project starts.
   b. The problem was identified and given a high priority by the nursing staff who would be affected by the change.

## Activity            10 MINUTES

Now return to the first activity in this subsection (p. 92) and see whether you would make any changes to your plan of action and chosen change.

## FEEDBACK

You may have identified a problem which is not seen as such by the staff and Reader Article 15 should have shown you that you are more likely to succeed if the staff feel that there is a problem. Also, have you fully considered the driving and resisting forces likely to be encountered?

Change is never achieved quickly, and it can backslide if momentum is lost, but the important thing is to keep on educating and try to win round more of

the waverers until the resistors find themselves in the minority, at which stage they have two choices, either to conform or leave.

## Self-assessment        15 MINUTES

1. Three different strategies might be used to achieve planned change. They are empirical rational, power coercive and normative educative. Underline the strategy which is most relevant to achieving change in a health care setting.
2. What are the six individual qualities a person needs to become a change agent as recognised by Wright?
3. What are the resistance/acceptance ranges you are likely to encounter from other people during the change process?

## FEEDBACK

1. You should have underlined normative re-educative as the most relevant change strategy for use in health care.

2. The individual qualities are:
   - possession of educational, managerial and clinical skills relevant to the area
   - proven communication skills both written and verbal
   - physical and psychological stamina
   - knowledge of how the health care system works
   - positive personal relationships outside work
   - commitment to the job.

3. You should have said: active resistance; passive resistance; apathy; passive acceptance; active acceptance.

## SUMMARY

Now that you have completed this section, you should know that:
- both patients and staff have rights and responsibilities relating to care
- requesting more resources requires a business plan and justification of why you are making your request
- changing practice takes time and commitment and must be carefully planned and implemented.

REFERENCES

Bernhard L, Walsh M 1981 Leadership—the key to the professionalisation of nursing. Allen Wayne Technical Group

Caldock K 1993 The Community Care White Paper—a nursing perspective. British Journal of Nursing 2(11): 592–597

Carpenter D 1992 Advocacy. Nursing Times 88(31)(suppl): 26–27

Clarke L 1994 Resource management in community nursing. District Nursing Association Newsletter (Spring): 16

Department of Health 1995 The Patients' Charter and you. Department of Health, London

Dimond B 1993 Patients' rights and responsibilities and the nurse. Quay Publishing, Lancaster

Griffiths R 1988 Community care agenda for action. HMSO, London

Niebuhr H R 1963 The responsible self. Harper & Row, New York

Teasdale K 1993 The case for change: implications of the caring for people White Paper. Professional Nurse 8(8): 543–545

Tingle J 1998 Nursing ethics and the law. Senior Nurse 8(2): 39–40

Tschudin V 1994 Deciding ethically. Baillière Tindall, London

UKCC 1992 Code of Professional Conduct for Nurses, Midwives and Health Visitors, revised edn. UKCC, London

Walsh M, Ford P 1989 Nursing rituals—research and rational actions. Heinemann Nursing, Oxford

Wright S 1985 Change in nursing. Nursing Practice 2: 85–91

Young A, Tingle J 1995 Record keeping. British Journal of Nursing 4(3): 179

FURTHER READING

Carnall C 1990 Managing change in organisations. Prentice Hall, Hemel Hempstead

Mabey C, Mayon-White (eds) 1993 Managing change. Paul Chapman Publishing, London

# A case history

The whole of this section is an activity intended to show whether or not you have understood some of the main issues relating to clinical care and pressure sores. It is based on Article 12 in the Reader (p. 147) and concerns the case of Mrs Jones, a patient who was admitted to hospital following a fall in which she fractured her femur. Following surgery and complications, a pressure sore began to develop which became progressively deeper. The article follows the treatment of her sore to eventual healing after 8 months.

Read the article, then, drawing on the knowledge you have gained from the preceding sections and Reader Articles, answer the questions given below.

1. List six predisposing factors which were present before or at the time of admission for this patient and say why they increase the risk of pressure sores.
2. List four factors which contributed to the formation of the pressure sore postoperatively, and say why.
3. Why do you think the pressure sore continued to deteriorate despite the different wound dressings used?
4. Chlorhexidine gauze was chosen as a dressing. Do you agree with the decision made? Give reasons for your answer.
5. What action does an airwave mattress have that reduces the effects of pressure? What are its claimed effects on the body which are said to speed up wound healing?
6. What is your reaction to the use of an incontinence sheet for the wound as opposed to dressings, once the patient was placed on the airwave mattress?
7. What did the care team learn as a result of this case?
8. Which of the team's costings suggest that they failed to learn some lessons from the case?
9. What do you consider were the main effects of this pressure sore for the patient?
10. List any policies, strategies, guidelines or personnel which would have helped this patient's care. For example you may think that a wound formulary would have prevented the inappropriate use of dressings.
11. If you had been involved in this case, how might you have used it to try to initiate some changes?

• • • • • • • • • • • • • • • • • • • • • • • • • • • • • • • • •

## FEEDBACK

1. The six predisposing factors which increased the risk of pressure sores were:

   • patient aged 68 years—studies show that those over 65 and the elderly ill are at high risk
   • fractured femur—which is identified as one of the highest risks especially when combined with age
   • muscle wasting—a cause of immobility and in itself one of the main causes of pressure sores because of the resulting pressure
   • urinary incontinence—increases the risk of maceration which will enhance the effect of shear forces
   • constipation—reducing nutritional intake, and leading to lethargy and immobility
   • depression—which may cause immobility and loss of appetite.

2. Four of the factors which contributed to pressure sore development postoperatively were as follows.

   • The patient was sat out in a chair every day, which results in high pressure to the sacrum.
   • Inappropriate pressure-relieving equipment was used—sheepskins, which do not relieve pressure, only shear and friction, and a foam overlay suitable for low-risk patients, or those being turned frequently.
   • There was no sense of urgency or prioritising of equipment even though a pressure sore was already developing.
   • There was no mention of reassessing the patient for risk, although this may have been done and not written down.

3. The pressure sore continued to develop because pressure was not removed. This was reinforced when the comment was made that the patient was easier to turn when the traction was

removed. Despite this, no pressure-relieving mattress was obtained over this critical period. It is also likely that the nutritional intake was inadequate, especially with the body attempting to heal a fracture and a pressure sore, but this was not mentioned. However, the very lack of mention indicates that a priority was not given to nutritional status.

4. Chlorhexidine tulle was not a suitable dressing choice because:

   • use of local antibacterials is not recommended for wound infections of this type
   • gauze is an unsuitable dressing for wounds because it fails to maintain the moist environment to aid healing, it can shed fibres into the wound, and it sticks to the wound bed.

5. The airwave is a pressure-relieving system which removes pressure from the body in an alternating cycle by inflating and deflating the cells under the patients. The timing of the cycle and the pressures achieved with the airwave system are said to promote flushing hyperaemia, which returns oxygen and nutrients to the tissues on removal of the high pressure.

6. Although the wound healed, use of an incontinence sheet indicated a lack of knowledge of the principles of wound healing and research-based practice. Its use between the patient and the mattress is not recommended. It is possible that the dry wound healing may have been painful, and the wound was exposed to risk of infection.

7. The team learnt that:

   • some dressings were harmful and their use was not backed up by research
   • suitable equipment was a vital part of prevention
   • failure to relieve the pressure to the sacrum was 'probably' the underlying cause
   • pressure relief should be available in chairs as well as beds.

8. Costings were looked at only in relation to purchase or rental of the mattress at a time when the patient had developed a pressure sore, and the suggestion was made that this cost would preclude widespread use in future. This is to totally ignore the following.

   • The cost of rental aimed at preventing the sore would have been less as the mattress would not have been needed for so long.
   • The total cost of 8 months' care for this patient because of the pressure sore, along with the reduced quality of life.

9. The main effects of the pressure sore for the patient were:

   • delayed discharge
   • inability to start mobilising
   • enforced bed rest

   and, although not mentioned, there may have been pain, social worries, a return of depression and distress from the smell of the wound.

10. It may be that policies and guidelines were in place but not being followed; however, the following would have helped the staff in this situation:

   • a wound formulary, to rationalise dressing choices and encourage research-based care
   • a flow chart to link risk assessment to equipment provision, tied in with standards relating to how soon this should be provided
   • a policy stressing all key areas such as nutrition, and supporting standards
   • a key person, link nurse or nurse specialist with knowledge which could have helped the staff.

11. This case could have been used for change in the following ways:

   • at ward level to improve ways patients are cared for by the whole team
   • by costing out the whole case financially, and presenting this to the management as an argument for providing more resources
   • by relating the care provided to quality of life issues and, with the financial costing, suggesting formation of a group to look at the problem in the unit or hospital.

## SUMMARY

This activity was aimed at pulling together some of the factors learnt throughout this pack. Hopefully it has reinforced:

• the importance of recognising the point at which a pressure sore begins, and taking immediate appropriate action relevant to that patient

• the significance of cost in terms of finance and costs to the patient's quality of life

• the fact that using traditional as opposed to research-based practice delays progress for the patient and can even be harmful

• the fact that a multidisciplinary policy and wound formulary may have helped in managing this patient, and provided a more structured approach to care.

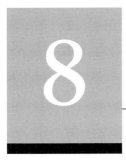

# 8 The future

This package has looked at what is happening in the field of pressure sores. It is likely that all nurses using it will have identified at least one area where practice in relation to pressure sores could be improved, showing that there is a need to move forward. The knowledge gained through this pack should have increased your awareness of the many and complex issues surrounding pressure sore prevention and management, and as with all learning this should now be used to improve patient care and quality of life. This section looks at what is happening now and some of the changes that are either underway or in the pipeline to implement moving forward.

## LEARNING OUTCOMES

At the end of this section, you should be able to:

- be aware of nurse prescribing and its implications
- identify the changes in health care delivery which have occurred
- identify ways of moving practice forward with particular relevance to your own area.

## 8.1 NATIONAL GUIDELINES

The NHS Executive has commissioned national guidelines on leg ulcer and pressure sore management, and these have been piloted in some areas. It was intended to discuss these in detail, but as yet they have not been released. Factors to consider when they do come out are whether they will be too prescriptive, not allowing for individual assessment and care as discussed in this pack. Additionally, as has been shown, if the guidelines require everyone to use one assessment tool or one grading system, this will invalidate much of the data already collected on the size of the pressure sore problem and necessitate re-education of staff who are not already using the advocated systems.

## 8.2 NURSE PRESCRIBING IN RELATION TO WOUND DRESSINGS

Throughout this pack you have learnt how to assess pressure sores and select dressings, and hopefully you

now feel confident to choose appropriate dressings to match this type of wound. The report by Baroness Cumberlege (DHSS 1986) recommended that there should be nurse prescribing for certain items and this now includes wound dressings. This section looks at the progress of nurse prescribing to date. It is important to note that the present recommendations only cover nursing staff with a community qualification, thus excluding some practice nurses and some community-based clinical nurse specialists.

Two reasons have been identified as to why the Cumberlege recommendations on nurse prescribing have not yet been implemented. These are:

- fears of rising costs
- the inevitable power struggle between some medical and nursing colleagues.

There are also concerns from pharmacists.

The reality of fears about costs is that there is no more money available to fund this initiative, and there will be several thousand more prescribers in the National Health Service if nurse prescribing goes ahead. Once again, the figure being looked at represents cost savings and not cost benefits, and it may well be necessary for nursing staff to measure this side of the equation, particularly if they wish to support their case. Edwards (1996) points out that in Wales alone over a 1-year period, prescribed wound management products came to £5.5 million. It is estimated that treating wounds costs £1 billion per annum nationally. There is no extra money available for nurse prescribing so costs will come out of this budget. For many years nurses have been advising medical staff on wound dressings, particularly in the community, and in effect prescribing them except that it has been the doctor's signature on the prescription and not that of the nurse. Pickersgill & Clarke (1990) identify this as a dangerous and confusing practice. In areas where multidisciplinary care is a reality, these decisions are often taken jointly. If nurses are to have the accountability of prescribing, they need to understand how best to use the wound products on the market, especially given the restrictions on FP10 as already discussed in Section 5.

They also need to understand the other aspects relating to wound healing, such as improving nutrition, so that dressings are not expected to be the miracle cure for a wound. Pickersgill & Clarke

(1990) cite the following as necessary for prescribing nurses:

1. the ability to undertake accurate assessments relating to individual patients within an holistic framework
2. the ability to explicitly justify decisions made
3. the ability to offer a range of treatment options other than pharmacological ones
4. the ability to evaluate treatments and revise decisions made if necessary.

The DoH Advisory Group on Nurse Prescribing (1989) recommended 3 days' additional training to prepare for the role of nurse prescriber. It is likely that this would be inadequate given the skills required and, in a small study of 28 district nurses, While & Rees (1993) found gaps in the nurses' knowledge that needed to be rectified, relating to both wound dressings and other factors relating to wound healing. It is likely that at least with some staff it would take longer than the 3 days recommended.

All articles relating to this subject stress how important education is before the project gets underway and as a prerequisite to being allowed to prescribe. A table by Britcair Ltd (1990) looks at present training and what would be needed to top it up also including clinical nurse specialists who work in the community in the equation. The irony of these educational recommendations is not lost on many nurses, when one considers the lack of wound care education given to medical staff who are presently responsible for prescribing, as highlighted by Bennett & Moody (1995). This education could be incorporated into future community nurse and specialist nurse training, allowing it to be given sufficient input to benefit staff.

Reasons why nurses should be able to prescribe wound care dressings are listed by Lockyer-Stevens & Bowden (1995) as follows:

- if a dressing is prescribed by a doctor, it could be applied by the nurse without correct wound assessment taking place
- doctors often prescribe dressings with which they are not familiar
- a nurse is not accountable for wound care, even though she/he will be applying dressings
- continuity of wound care might be disrupted
- dressings might be applied according to availability rather than appropriateness
- treatment delays may occur while waiting for a doctor to prescribe dressings.

Howard (1996) and Gething (1996) give two different views on nurse prescribing. To look at the effects of nurse prescribing, eight pilot sites were selected by the DoH at GP fund holding practices around the country and 62 nurses trained to become

nurse prescribers. Nurses were issued with different coloured prescription pads so that their prescriptions could be easily identified. A survey in May 1995 after 6 months (Editorial 1995) showed:

- patients got prescriptions more quickly
- nurses felt they were delivering a complete package of care instead of part of one
- nurses showed increased confidence in their work
- cost was not mentioned.

**Activity**    20 MINUTES

Article 16 in the Reader (p. 160) gives an overview of the nurses' formulary and benefits to practice. Having read this article, answer the following questions.

1. In the Cumberlege report, what were the two main issues which led to the concept of nurse prescribing?
2. When using the nurse prescribers' formulary, which other publication should be referred to, particularly if prescribing wound care products?
3. What benefits are identified for the patients in nurse prescribing?

**FEEDBACK**

1. The two main issues identified in the Cumberlege report were as follows.

   a. Much time is spent by patients, carers and district nurses in obtaining prescriptions.
   b. Nurses often have more expertise in the use of prescribed products than doctors.

2. You should have said that the British National Formulary (BNF) should be used as well when prescribing dressings.

3. The following are identified as benefits to patients:

   a. improved patient care because of the nurses' ability to prescribe items meeting the nursing needs of the patient
   b. informed discussion with the patient about suitable treatments and appliances
   c. quicker treatment decisions, because the nurse can work independently.

Lockyer-Stevens & Bowden (1995) described an initiative to allow nurse prescribing in the hospital sector and reported on problems encountered, the majority of which could be put down to lack of education and limited range of dressings used. They also reported that nurse prescribing can lead to better continuity of wound care, and that expenditure in hospital did not rise as a result.

Once again, the key to success would appear to lie with education. Additionally, a wound formulary, especially across care boundaries, would help rationalise decision making and promote continuity of care. It also needs cost benefits as opposed to cost expenditure to be considered in the final equation.

### Self-assessment    15 MINUTES

1. Whose report initiated nurse prescribing?
2. Who can prescribe?
3. How can nurses be educated for nurse prescribing?

• • • • • • • • • • • • • • • • • • • • • • • • • • • • • •

### FEEDBACK

1. The report which initiated nurse prescribing was by Baroness Cumberlege (DHSS 1986).
2. Nurses with community qualifications who have received extra training can prescribe. There are moves afoot to include specialist nurses who work in the community.
3. Nurses will have training incorporated into their basic training, and for those qualified now there are ENB packs and videos.

• • • • • • • • • • • • • • • • • • • • • • • • • • • • • •

## 8.3 CHANGES IN CARE DELIVERY

The Griffiths report (1988) laid the foundation for the present health care changes. There is no denying that some change was necessary, and that there had been some waste of resources. According to Ranade (1994) the Conservative Government has seen the following changes:

- greater fragmentation of service delivery
- commitment to competition
- the purchaser/provider split
- more options, e.g. commercial, voluntary and informal care provision
- consumer choice, the Patients' Charter
- attempts to shift power from the unions and the power groups, e.g. doctors
- commercial style management for welfare agencies
- accountability including targets and monitoring of results.

These changes have been rushed through with little in the way of pilot work to assess their effectiveness, although there is a school of thought that this was the only way to inflict change on such a huge bureaucratic machinery as the NHS. The main change affecting everyone is the purchaser/provider split and most of the others result from this.

### Self-assessment    10 MINUTES

From your existing knowledge who would you identify as:

1. purchasers?
2. providers?

• • • • • • • • • • • • • • • • • • • • • • • • • • • • • •

### FEEDBACK

You should have identified that the district health authorities (DHA) or commissioning agencies and the GP fund holders are the main purchasers and the individual trusts now formed are the providers, whether they are acute hospitals, community trusts or a combination of both.

• • • • • • • • • • • • • • • • • • • • • • • • • • • • • •

The role of the purchasers is to obtain the best care on behalf of the patient (who is the consumer), and additionally in the case of the DHA and GPs to assess the health needs for their population. Providers are expected to give value for money and be more accountable for the quality of care provided and the costs involved. This has already been discussed in Section 6. 25% of the NHS budget is related to nursing services, and 80% of direct patient care is provided by nurses, midwives and health visitors (CDNA 1994). An effective way of showing cost improvement is in rationalisation of nursing services, usually by looking at skill mix, and many nurses will have been subjected to this, particularly in hospitals. Unfortunately this does not ensure quality care, and there have already been articles in the press decrying the lack of nursing care being provided. In the community, different models for managing community nursing services are emerging. Reid & David (1994) give examples of some of these models in practice.

Benson (1995) identifies primary care-led purchasing and the opportunities for nurses to move into purchasing to influence what is happening in the health care market today. He also makes the point that nurse education needs to change to produce new nurses with the ability to think. It is unlikely that the public are aware of all the changes which are occurring, and this is another reason that nurses must fight to be involved in health care changes and decisions.

Fragmentation of care, as quoted earlier, is also a major problem. Since April 1993 and as a direct consequence of the White Paper *Caring for People* (Secretaries of State for Health, 1989), social services have had the responsibility for assessing social care needs, while health care staff are supposed to continue to assess and plan for health care needs. In complex cases, care managers will be appointed to oversee individual patients and coordinate care. This system was set up on the assumption that people would work together, but as Hudson (1992) says, there is little evidence to show that this has ever occurred. Certainly the speed with which the changes were introduced gave little time for communication and network pathways to be built. An additional problem is that social services do not always recognise a nursing need when they assess patients, and so district nurses are not involved. This is particularly true where the risk of pressure sores occurs. More education needs to be given to staff and assessors on health aspects, or district nurses need to be routinely asked about patients being assessed so that they can do a nursing assessment at the same time.

Although the idea was that collaboration and consultation between agencies would occur, this is not the reality. Article 14 in the Reader gives a case study where a patient developed a pressure sore because of problems in the total care package.

---

**Activity**      **15 MINUTES**

Read the case history in Reader Article 14 (p. 154) and suggest two failures in care planning which contributed to the breakdown of care.

• • • • • • • • • • • • • • • • • • • • • • • • • • • • •

## FEEDBACK

You should have said the following.

1. There was no collaboration between health and social care workers.
2. The patient's needs were not central to the package of care.

• • • • • • • • • • • • • • • • • • • • • • • • • • • • •

Unfortunately this is not an isolated incident and, coupled with the fact that social services receive money for social care and health authorities for health care, the issue is what is deemed health care and what social care. This has led, in some areas, to resentments

between agencies which affect patient care. Providing sufficient resources in the community is the job of the health purchasers, but to do this they need to know about unmet need, knowledge which can be provided by nursing staff. Joint committees do exist in some areas, and are beginning to emerge more now, but these should have been in place, along with dialogue between the two groups, before the reforms were introduced. As Elliott points out in her article (Reader 14), two different organisational cultures are involved here, along with all the usual problems related to change.

## 8.4 THE WAY FORWARD

The purpose of this pack has been to show what needs to be done to improve prevention and management of pressure sores and give food for thought within your own work areas about aspects which could be improved. To make improvements, nurses need to be proactive. Given briefly below are some issues to think about in relation to moving the prevention and management of pressure sores forward in your area.

### Standard setting

It is not the place of this pack to cover standard setting in terms of how to do it, as all nurses should have the knowledge to do this now. It is, however, important to remember why we have standards; they are a measure against which to judge nursing performance. This is not synonymous with effective outcomes, for example terminal care patients will die, but this does not prevent setting standards in relation to their care. Standards should always be set with patients as their central theme (Watkins 1991) and, providing they do this, they can also be used to identify service expectations to patients and purchasers of health care.

Standards should be:

- explicit—that is, people trying to work to them know what is expected of them
- measurable—to see if they are being achieved
- achievable—not hampered by influences over which people have no control
- realistic—relevant to the situation.

---

**Activity**      **40 MINUTES**

1. Identify three standards in use in your area, one each relating to:

  - risk assessment
  - prevention of pressure sores
  - treatment of pressure sores.

2.  In Table 8.1, write down in the columns whether each standard meets the criteria.

If no standards have been set in your area, write one for each of the categories in Question 1 and check whether they meet the criteria in Table 8.1.

. . . . . . . . . . . . . . . . . . . . . . . . . . . . . . . . . . . .

## FEEDBACK

Your answer will depend very much on your own area. In the unlikely event that you had no standard the ones you have set should be agreed with your colleagues and should be introduced as quickly as possible. Examples might be as follows.

**Risk assessment.** All patients will be assessed for risk of pressure sore development within 2 hours of admission to hospital or nursing home. In the community this should be done during the first visit by qualified nursing staff.

**Prevention of pressure sores.** All patients assessed as being at high risk of pressure sore development to have a pressure-relieving mattress in situ within 2 hours of assessment. In the community this may read to have a plan of care for turning and moving the patient in situ within 2 hours of risk assessment.

**Treatment of pressure sores.** All patients recognised as having pressure damage to have the sore graded and measured at the time the sore is first recorded and appropriate treatment instigated.

All three of these statements are explicit, achievable and realistic but unless documentation is correctly filled in, they cannot be measured. For example, times will need to be filled in for assessment and provision of equipment, as was shown in Section 6.1, correct documentation is essential, and this is another area where it really counts. An audit of assessment times that showed a shortfall of identifying patients at risk may point the way to reducing the incidence of pressure sores by early recognition and taking preventive measures in time to prevent damage occurring.

. . . . . . . . . . . . . . . . . . . . . . . . . . . . . . . . . . . .

## Audit

Again, the key considerations only will be given. Audit is very much the 'buzz word' at present and is often held up as a measure of quality. It is, however, important to remember that while it often identifies areas of practice which can be improved, especially against set standards, it does not always measure the quality of care or life. An example of this is the standard relating to risk assessment. Measured on its own it will tell you whether the standard is being met but it will not tell you whether any action is being taken with regard to the risk scores achieved. Audit can be done on small areas such as a single standard or larger ones, where problems identified may show the way forward to improving care. It can also be done by asking patients and staff or retrospectively by looking at nursing and medical records. People planning to do an audit involving direct patient contact will have to take it to an audit committee at the planning stage for agreement to continue.

| Table 8.1 | | | | |
|---|---|---|---|---|
| Standard | Is it explicit? | Is it measurable? | Is it achievable? | Is it realistic? |
|  |  |  |  |  |

## Activity     45 MINUTES

Article 17 in the Reader (p. 163) is useful at this stage because it covers so many areas discussed in this package, and pulls them together. It describes an audit done of community hospitals in the Grampian region with varying clientele.

1. Read the article, then list under the following four headings what was found in the audit.

   - Risk assessment, for example some patients were not assessed for risk
   - Pressure sores
   - Dressings
   - Prevention.

2. Write down the actions taken following the audit and say whether they have been suggested in this pack.

● ● ● ● ● ● ● ● ● ● ● ● ● ● ● ● ● ● ● ● ● ● ● ● ● ● ● ● ●

## FEEDBACK

1. You should have identified the following under the various headings.

   - Risk assessment:
     —some patients not assessed
     —some wards not using a risk assessment tool
     —some patients not identified as at risk still developed pressure sores.

   - Pressure sores:
     —the data on where the sore started was not always recorded
     —a high number of buttock sores suggested that patients were sitting out for too long.

   - Dressings:
     —most were chosen by the nurses, but not always appropriately
     —there were many different regimes for dressings.

   - Prevention:
     —there was a shortfall of the right sort of equipment
     —some equipment needed repairing.

2. The outcome of the audit was that:

   - a multidisciplinary team was formed
   - link nurses from across boundaries were brought together
   - a policy has been drafted
   - a monthly prevalence audit has been set up.

All of these have been mentioned in this pack as the way forward. Think of your own area, and whether you could do all or a part of this audit. Would you be able to evaluate whether the correct equipment was provided for a patient? Do you know if all your patients have been assessed for risk?

● ● ● ● ● ● ● ● ● ● ● ● ● ● ● ● ● ● ● ● ● ● ● ● ● ● ● ● ● ●

In addition to all that you have learned so far, for successful change to take place there needs to be an appropriate climate for change, otherwise new initiatives may not succeed. Again education and link nurses can lead the way in this.

## Research and/or evaluation of care

This can provide a more comprehensive look at care and often provides better quality indicators in relation to quality of life issues. To undertake research you will need to take your proposal to the ethics committee. Suggestions for areas to look at could include:

- effectiveness of equipment as discussed in Section 4
- cost benefit as opposed to cost effectiveness
- quality of life issues.

## Activity     1 HOUR

In your own area identify one topic which you would like to know more about, and write down how you could set about gaining this information.

● ● ● ● ● ● ● ● ● ● ● ● ● ● ● ● ● ● ● ● ● ● ● ● ● ● ● ● ● ●

## FEEDBACK

This will depend on you. If you wish to know where the majority of pressure sores in your care setting started, then you will need to audit all the patients' notes to find this information, unless you already have a monitoring system in place. If you want to find out how a pressure sore has affected a patient's quality of life, you will need to devise a questionnaire such as was covered in Section 2. What is important is that you start to do something, so that the knowledge you have gained through studying is passed on and benefits the patients in your care.

● ● ● ● ● ● ● ● ● ● ● ● ● ● ● ● ● ● ● ● ● ● ● ● ● ● ● ● ● ●

## SUMMARY

Now that you have completed this section, you should know that:

- for nurse prescribing to be effective, nurses must be able to justify their choice of wound care dressings
- nurses need to become more proactive in the new health care environment, particularly if they wish to continue to do the best for their patients
- identifying an area for improvement in your own area is the way to start moving forward.

## REFERENCES

Bennett G, Moody M 1995 Wound care for health professionals. Chapman & Hall, London

Benson D 1995 Opportunity or threat? Nursing Standard 9(22): 22–23

Britcair Ltd 1990 Educating for change. Nursing Standard 4(44): 13–14

Community District Nursing Association (CDNA) 1994 Building a stronger team. Nursing Care (Autumn): 5

Department of Health and Social Security 1986 Neighbourhood nursing: a focus for care. Report of the Community Nursing Review (Chairman: Julia Cumberlege) HMSO, London

Department of Health 1989 Report of the Advisory Group on Nurse Prescribing. HMSO, London

Editorial 1995 Nurse prescribing demonstration sites are successful. Nurse Prescriber (May): 3

Edwards L 1996 Reality and the drug tariff. Nursing Care (Winter 95/96): 13

Gething A 1996 The non-prescriber. Nursing Notes 11(March): 5

Griffiths R 1988 Community care agenda for action. HMSO, London

Howard B 1996 The prescriber. Nursing Notes 11(March): 4

Hudson R 1992 Ignorance and apathy. Health Service Journal (March): 24–25

Lockyer-Stevens N, Bowden J 1995 Nurse prescribing of wound care dressings. Professional Nurse 10(11): 697–702

Pickersgill F, Clarke S 1990 A prescription for nursing. Nursing Standard 4(44): 10–11

Ranade W 1994 A future for the NHS? Longman Group UK, London

Reid T, David A 1994 Community nursing practice management and teamwork. Nursing Times 90(51): 42–45

Secretaries of State for Health, Wales and Scotland 1989 Caring for people. Cmnd 849. HMSO, London

Watkins M 1991 Nursing knowledge ultimate objectives. In: Perry A, Jolley M (eds) Nursing—a knowledge base for practice. Edward Arnold, Kent

While A, Rees K 1993 Prescribing potential. Journal of Wound Care Nursing 89(48): 1–4

# Reader

# Prevalence of pressure damage in hospital patients in the UK

K. O'Dea, SRN, RMN, FETCert, is product manager, clinical services, Support Systems International, Solihull

## Results

### Overall prevalence rates

Some 3 213 adult in-patients were seen over a one-year period (only three refused permission). Five hundred and ninety eight of these patients had pressure damage, which included those with persistent non-blanching hyperaemia. This gives an overall prevalence rate of 18.6%, with a range of 22.8% to 14.4%. The mean prevalence, excluding non-blanching hyperaemia (stage 1), was 10.1%, range 11.6% to 8.6%.

### Severity of pressure damage

The largest variation occurred in the proportion of damaged areas which were full-thickness wounds (stage 3, 4 and those in which eschar was present). It is these wounds that indicated a failure of prevention strategies. The highest proportion (that is, the percentage of damaged areas which were full-thickness wounds) was 30%, and the lowest was 11%, with a mean of 20% (Fig 5). Further analysis indicates that 3.6% of all the hospital in-patients had a full-thickness pressure sore. Patients had an average of 1.7 wounds each.

### The patients

Females made up 63% of all hospital patients and 59% of the pressure damage group. Analysis of the combined age data revealed that 1 435 (44%) out of a total of 3 213 patients were over 70 years. Individual hospitals varied in the percentage of their patients over 70 years; the highest being a teaching hospital (51.9%). That hospital also had the lowest overall prevalence rate

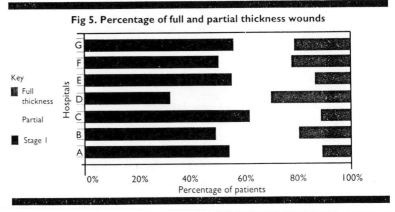

Fig 5. Percentage of full and partial thickness wounds

Key
■ Full thickness
Partial
■ Stage I

(14.4%). The lowest incidence of over-70s (34.3%) was in a district general hospital. Patients with pressure damage were more likely to be over 70 years, but again this varied. In one teaching hospital with a high prevalence (21.2%), only 42.8% of pressure damage patients were over 70 years, but of the 598 patients with damage from all the studies, 66.4% were over 70 years.

### Risk scores
Of the 3 213 patients, 32% scored over 15 on the Waterlow Scale (that is, they had a high risk of developing pressure damage). This was fairly consistent throughout all the hospitals with less than half of all in-patients falling into a 'no risk' category (Fig 6).

### Source of damage
The highest rate of hospital-acquired damage was 80% of the total (occurring in a teaching hospital) with the lowest 51% (in a district general hospital). The mean was 68.2%. All patients admitted to hospital with damage had a higher proportion of full-thickness stage 3 and 4 wounds and those with eschar (Figs 7 and 8).

### Support surfaces
Most patients were nursed on an ordinary hospital mattress. The next most commonly used surface was a fibre-filled overlay on which 12% of all patients were nursed. Some 33% of patients with pressure damage and 31% with a risk score of more than 20 were nursed on a standard hospital mattress. There was no direct relationship between the patients' risk score, or pressure area condition, and the chosen support surface.

### Documentation
Of the 598 patients with damage, 52% had a care plan relating to either treatment or prevention. A further 27% received a mention

at some point in the nursing records but 21% had no nursing documentation relating to pressure damage. Medical notes were not examined.

### Discussion
This study shows a high prevalence of pressure damage (18.6%) in contrast to the published DoH figure of 6.7%[3]. Excluding stage 1 damage (persistent non-blanching hyperaemia), which some authors ignore, there still remains a prevalence of 10.1%. It is important to recognise that, while stage 1 damage must be taken into account, it can distort the figures. For example, a hospital with a high overall prevalence but with a low prevalence of stage 2 to 4 wounds indicates that prevention strategies are to some degree effective.

The prevalence of pressure damage bore no relation to hospital type, and the findings show similar trends in all seven hospitals. The figures confirm that there is an increased risk of pressure damage in elderly patients (66.4% being over 70 years) but this is by no means confined to that age group, around one-third of the patients with damage being under 70 years. Also, a high proportion of elderly patients did not necessarily result in a high prevalence.

The Waterlow risk assessment tool was used in all seven hospitals and was the tool chosen by them to provide a profile of patients at varying degrees of risk. Often, use of the tool formed part of the hospital policy on the prevention of pressure damage. It is reasonable to conclude from the figures that around one-third of all in-patients should have in place a care plan including all aspects of prevention of pressure damage. In fact only 52% of patients with established damage had such a care plan.

The results indicate that almost 70% of damaged areas developed while patients were in the care of the hospital. However, that does leave a substantial number who were admitted from various sources. The patients admitted with damage, while fewer in number, did tend to have a higher proportion of full thickness wounds (Figs 7 and 8). This was a consistent finding in all the hospitals and is important information for those planning treatment and prevention protocols. Internal hospital policies that aim at reducing the development of pressure damage will not impact on this particular group and provision must be made for them. A redesigned data collection tool now in print will enable us to identify the source of admission. One author[6] stated that the separation of hospital-acquired sores and those present on admission is an essential part of clinical audit and quality

6 Richardson, B. Hospital versus community-acquired pressure sores: should prevalence rates be separated? *J Tissue Viability* 1993; **3**: 13–15.

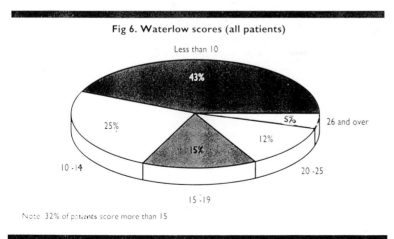

**Fig 6. Waterlow scores (all patients)**

Less than 10 — 43%

26 and over — 5%

20 -25 — 12%

15 -19 — 15%

10 -14 — 25%

Note: 32% of patients score more than 15

assurance, and also remarked on the high proportion of stage 3 and 4 wounds in the admitted group.

Many different support surfaces were in use, but availability was more often the criteria for choice rather than the patients' needs. Many written hospital policies base the criteria for choosing a support surface on the risk score of the patient, but in practice there is no close correlation between the two[5]. The reasons for this needs to be more fully explored. It may be that risk score alone provides insufficient information for the choice of support system, or it may be that a patient meets certain criteria but support surfaces are denied because of budget constraints or lack of knowledge.

It is likely that a combination of these factors, and perhaps others, are at work. That different levels of support system have different pressure-relieving characteristics is well documented and the cost of using support systems must be balanced against the cost of failing to use them appropriately.

The most striking finding on examining all the information from these surveys is the lack of a systematic approach to pressure damage prevention and treatment, even when lengthy protocols had been produced. This was indicated by the low priority given to documenting a care plan for prevention and treatment. This, of course, does not mean that nurses were not giving conscientious care to those patients at risk, but in many cases they would have been unable to show that they had planned care, given that care and evaluated its effectiveness.

### Conclusions and recommendations

Previously, prevalence of pressure damage has been quoted as being anything between 3.0 and 94%. The lack of comparability of data that led to the use of a percentage range rather than a specific number was owing to the differing methodologies and definitions used. It should now be possible to use these figures as a benchmark and to begin to make comparisons between different surveys not only in the UK but internationally. A multi-site survey in the USA in 1989 using almost identical methodology and involving 148 hospitals and 34 987 patients yielded an overall prevalence rate of 9.2%[7]. In 1992, as yet unpublished surveys of three German hospitals (2 172 patients) showed an overall prevalence of 15.6%.

An enormous amount has been written about the phenomenon of pressure damage, particularly over the past five years. The Health of the Nation and a report by the National Audit Office[8] indicate that the problem is a management issue. This can only be helpful in

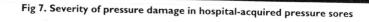

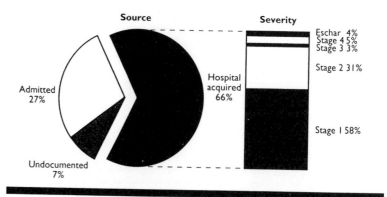

**Fig 7. Severity of pressure damage in hospital-acquired pressure sores**

Source

Admitted 27%

Undocumented 7%

Hospital acquired 66%

Severity

Eschar 4%
Stage 4 5%
Stage 3 3%
Stage 2 31%
Stage 1 58%

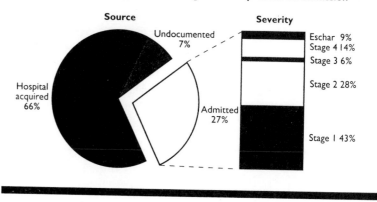

**Fig 8. Severity of pressure damage in sores present on admission**

Source

Undocumented 7%

Hospital acquired 66%

Admitted 27%

Severity

Eschar 9%
Stage 4 14%
Stage 3 6%
Stage 2 28%
Stage 1 43%

the establishment of effective policies which close the gap between theory and practice. Such policies must use valid and reliable information as a first step, followed by active implementation which monitors the outcomes, balancing quality and cost.

This article does not include every aspect of the data collected, but the surveys we have carried out indicate that the size of the problem is greater than has hitherto been assumed. The generalisability of the data is limited to a certain extent, as all these hospitals had an active interest in the problem and a desire to improve things. They also had in common an enthusiastic and committed staff, an openness about this thorny problem and a willingness to work collaboratively with SSI.

Our experience has indicated improvements which we can make to the data collection and analysis. New forms and software have been produced, and a larger database will allow more detailed analysis to be performed. We would welcome constructive comments and suggestions on how to improve this unique service, which sets a new standard for this aspect of audit. ∎

7 Meehan, M. Multisite pressure ulcer prevalence survey. *Decubitus* 1989; **3**: 4, 14–17.
8 National Audit Office. *Health Services for Physically Disabled People Aged 16–64.* London: HMSO, 1992.

# NUTRITION AND WOUND HEALING

G. Pinchcofsky-Devin, RD, FACN, vice-president, enteral services, Stat Homecare, Elmhurst, Illinois, USA

## PROTEIN

Protein is an essential nutrient for healing. The normal serum albumin concentration is 35–50g/l in the serum of the adult. This level is the equilibrium point between the production, distribution and degradation of albumin. The skin represents 30–40% of the extravascular albumin stores.

Albumin catabolism increases as a result of injury to the skin as does other plasma protein catabolism. Albumin is made available to regeneration tissue in proportion to the extent of injury and inflammation. Changes in temperature and pH at the injury site denature the native albumin. Macrophages are then able to utilise the constituents of the albumin.

Serum albumin in the wounded patient falls. If severe such a decrease in serum albumin synthesis or increase in albumin utilisation at a major wound site may impair wound healing in the patient.

As metabolic stress increases with injury, infection or open wounds the body uses protein as a greater portion of the total energy expenditure. Intake should increase to 1.5 to 2.5g/kg daily to avoid negative nitrogen balance and place the patient in a state of anabolism. With pressure sores healing can be achieved only with a high-protein diet. Providing adequate fluid for the patient is essential.

There is a clear correlation between the patient's dietary intake of protein and the development of pressure sores.

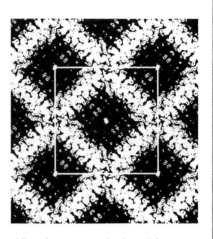

**Albumin: computerised model**

## NUTRITIONAL ASSESSMENT

Early identification and monitoring of several nutrition risk factors may eliminate or reduce the complications associated with delayed wound healing. These nutrition risk factors include:
- Decreased serum albumin level below 35g/l
- Low serum transferrin level below 1800mg/l
- Low total lymphocyte count below 1800 cells/mm³
- Anemia; haemoglobin below 12mg/dl
- Decreased oral intake.

The nutrition risk factors can be identified by performing a nutritional assessment.

The three major components of nutritional assessment are the visceral protein stores, the somatic protein stores and the vitamin and mineral status of the patient.

## TRACE ELEMENTS

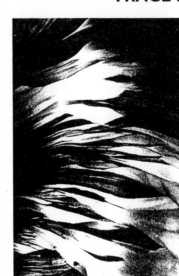

**Zinc: polarised light micrograph**

Zinc is needed for the transcription of RNA in the promotion of protein synthesis, cellular replication and collagen formation. Zinc deficiency has an adverse influence on wound healing through its effect on reducing rates of epithelialisation, decreasing of wound strength and collagen synthesis.

Iron is necessary for the hydroxylation of lysine and proline in the formation of collagen. Iron is necessary to transport oxygen in the body.

Copper is necessary for collagen cross-link formation. Together with iron, copper is essential to the production of erythrocytes.

Poor nutrition can contribute to the development of chronic wounds, such as pressure sores or surgical wounds, in several ways.

A diet deficient in many nutrients, particularly those involved in protein synthesis, jeopardises tissue integrity and contributes to skin breakdown. In addition, inadequate caloric intake causes weight loss and a reduction in subcutaneous tissue, allowing bony prominences to compress and restrict circulation to the skin. The resultant reduction of the nutrients supplied to that area also promotes tissue catabolism.

The three steps in the healing response involve and are dependent on nutritional substrates: These steps are:
■ Inflammation with recruitment of polymorphonuclear leukocytes, macrophages and lymphocytes
■ The proliferation of fibroblasts and the production of collagen
■ Collagen remodelling and re-epithelialisation when appropriate.

The strength and integrity of tissue repair will depend on collagen cross-linking and deposition.

# CARBOHYDRATE AND FATS

Carbohydrates and fats provide a source of cellular energy. Glucose, the simplest form of carbohydrate, is the primary fuel for cellular metabolism of many tissues, including leukocytes, fibroblasts and macrophages. When glucose is not available for cellular function, the body catabolises protein and, to a lesser degree, fat, to produce glucose to meet energy requirements. Glucose is needed to meet the metabolic demand for wound healing and preserve the body's structural and functional protein.

Energy from fat metabolism is used in all normal cell functions, and fat metabolism results in the formation of prostaglandins and other regulators of the immune and inflammatory process.

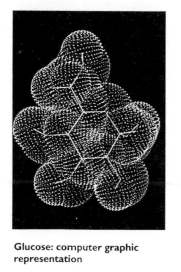

**Glucose: computer graphic representation**

# VITAMINS

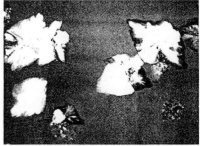

**Vitamin A: dietary sources include butter, egg yolks and fish liver oils**

**Vitamin C: water soluble, found in fresh fruit and vegetables**

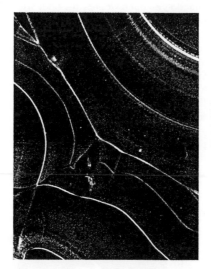

The natural process of wound healing requires numerous energy-consuming reactions and these all require increased amounts of vitamins. Where specific vitamin deficiencies are diagnosed, individual supplements of up to 10 to 20 times the recommended daily allowance may be needed. Supplementation is an extremely important component of the therapeutic nutrition care plan for the patient with a wound.

Vitamin C functions as a co-factor in the hydroxylation of proline to hydroxyproline, an essential step in the synthesis of collagen. Vitamin C deficiency markedly delays the wound-healing process and causes capillary fragility. In vitamin C deficiency states, old wounds may re-open because of loss of tensile strength and degeneration of the extracellular matrix.

Ascorbic acid may increase the activation of leukocytes and macrophages to the injured site.

Vitamin A is important in maintaining the normal humoral defence mechanism and in limiting complications associated with wound infections either locally or systemically. Supplementation of retinoic acid has been shown to improve wound healing in patients receiving corticosteroid treatment.

Vitamin A is required for an adequate inflammatory response, which is essential for the formation of mucopolysaccharides. These function as a protective sheath around collagen. The supplementation of vitamin A in steroid-dependent patients before surgery may promote a rapid healing response and reduce the incidence of wound dehiscence.

Vitamin E is essential for the stability of cell walls. Decreased levels of vitamin E are associated with shortened survival of red and white blood cells. Vitamin E also enhances the immune response. Vitamin K plays an essential role in coagulation, which is a prerequisite for healing.

# Maintaining Nutritional Support in the Community

## Elizabeth Oliver

*Manager, Nutrition and Dietetics*
*Milton Keynes General Hospital*

A paper presented at the 21st Conference of the Society, Bristol

The scope of the topic is very wide so I have broken it down into three areas:

1 Who are we feeding and why?

2 What are we feeding and how?

3 Some practical problems

I will also try to mention in passing the other professionals involved as this is very much a multi-disciplinary problem.

## 1 WHO ARE WE FEEDING AND WHY?

In the context of wound healing, food has two essential functions.

Firstly, it provides raw materials for repairing the wound and secondly, good nutrition is essential to ensure a well functioning immune system. It is ironic that in the third world these two facts are readily appreciated and when we see hungry people on the news, it is obvious that they are not really going to get well whilst they are still hungry. (We know for example that measles is a far more serious problem to children in the third world than it is here) yet we seem to forget in our hi-tech health care system that the same applies to us.

The report *A Positive Approach to Nutrition as Treatment* published by the King's Fund Centre in January 1992, gives a very good overview of nutritional problems both in hospitals and in the community. It talks about resources and costs and other relevant points, some of which I shall cover later.

### What are the effects of malnutrition on somebody who is ill?

Malnutrition leads to a downward spiral of worsening health and quality of life. In Table 1, the first three points – poor concentration, apathy, and depression – not only lead to a very negative approach to getting well, but of particular relevance in this context, they are likely to reduce the desire to eat. Reduced food intake leads to loss of muscle power, including the respiratory muscles. If you cannot cough then you are more prone to chest infections and you are back to compromising your nutritional status and the ability to fight infection.

| | |
|---|---|
| Inability to concentrate | |
| Apathy | |
| Depression | |
| Impaired Appetite | |
| Loss of muscle power – | Respiratory Cardiac problems |
| Mobility Reduced – | Thromboembolism Pressure sores |
| Reduced immunocompetence – Infection | |
| Altered structure and function – Malabsorption of gut | |

Table 1 Effects of Malnutrition

The loss of muscle power also means that your mobility is reduced, which is a factor in pressure sore prevention. If you are not very mobile, your rehabilitation is impaired and that also includes your ability to get out, shop, cook and feed yourself. The unkindest thing of all is that if you are starving then your gut is starved. You fail to absorb all your food and the downward spiral starts again.

### Who in the community needs help?

Table 2 is a list of the types of people in the local community at present to whom my department gives nutritional support. Part of the process of maintaining nutrition within the community is to go out and make your own list of people in need. It will be similar but will vary with different populations. I advise this quite glibly but I know that it may be difficult to find out who needs help. Having tried to start an audit of sufferers from dysphagia due to CVA we are finding the most difficult part is deciding where to start and who to approach.

The categories in Table 2 actually overlap and a patient may well fit more than one category. I am going to start with the elderly and frail because they are the largest group and are very prone to pressure sores. Their problems may well apply to the other categories.

| Elderly |
| --- |
| CVA |
| MS/MND |
| Cancers |
| Dysphagia |

Table 2  Who is at risk?

**What factors affect nutrition in the elderly?**
Some of the relevant factors are listed in Table 3.

**Money** – There may be real problems with money because the pension doesn't go very far, or with problems of perception of values and resources. If your mind is wandering back 20 or 30 years then today's prices seem horrendous.

**Loneliness** – Nobody sits down to eat a nice plate full of proteins and vitamins. They eat **food** which is appetizing and pleasant and is better if there is somebody to share the meal with you.

**Physical ability** – In the wider sense this means the ability to get out and do the shopping. Sometimes you have to look beyond nutrition itself to things like geography and transport. In Milton Keynes, which is very flat and also has fairly good community transport, perhaps this particular problem is deferred longer than in a rural area which is hilly and has poor community transport.

**Physical ability to cook is a relevant factor** – Can you cook safely? Can you lift a full pan of boiling water? Occupational Therapists are particularly useful in assessing what is needed and for devising aids for steadying kettles and so on. Do you actually have the dexterity to feed yourself? Can you manage to get the food into your mouth and not around your ears?

Also relevant to this problem are means of care and support. The sort of care and support that you get from Care Assistants was discussed this morning. When your family are the carers their help may depend on their other commitments so that, if you are elderly, your ability to get access to food may well depend on what sort of job your daughter-in-law does and how easily she can get home at lunch time to feed you.

**Confusion** – This raises questions such as: Did you remember to eat? Did you remember what to open and how to cook it? Silly things like do your teeth fit and is this altering what you chose to eat? Something we do not like to mention is incontinence, which may be linked to mobility. If you cannot get to the loo in time, then you may cut out all those cups of tea, together with a lot of the meal supplements that are in liquid form. Then you will not be taking all that the dietician suggests, causing problems later on, because of reduced nutritional intake.

| Financial | | |
| --- | --- | --- |
| Depression/Loneliness | | |
| Physical Abilities | To Shop | |
| | To Cook | |
| | To Eat | |
| Acceptance | | |
| Carer Support | | |
| Confusion | | |
| Teeth/Indigestion | | |
| Continence | | |

Table 3  Factors Affecting Nutritional Intake

The COMA report 1992 from *The Nutrition of Elderly People* covers many of these problems.

**How does one actually find out which individuals are at risk?**
In the community, how do we identify the people with problems? In fact the problems may be quite insidious and nothing really shows until perhaps a crisis precipitates investigation. The over-75 screening may provide an inroad, but for the young elderly and those with other problems, how do we go about finding out what the problems are?

Dr Louise Davis from the Royal Free, devised a useful grid for identifying those who may have problems. This is shown in Table 4. Across the top you have risk factors, e.g. loneliness, depression etc. You select the relevant ones. Against those are plotted warning signals. When the two come together, you have a situation which should really initiate further investigation. Another way is to use a screening system, perhaps your own which you have made relevant to the population you are looking after.

Referring again to Table 2, the next group of concern was those with CVA. They share the problems of the elderly. Most of them are elderly. In addition they may have a swallowing problem which will lead firstly to a reduced food intake and secondly may cause them to aspirate some of their food which in turn may lead to a chest infection. The nice thing (if one can put it that way) about CVA is that providing you do not have a second one or extend the ones you've got the dysphagia often improves. Not so those with neurological problems. This group is usually younger, they may well have dysphagia, they may lose manual dexterity and they have a progressive disorder. To have worsening problems with food is inevitable and that is demoralising. The food tends to become a bit of a benchmark as to how you're progressing so these are the people who deny there is a problem and resist attempts to assist. This has to be tackled with a great deal of sensitivity, whilst still hoping ultimately to get the desired result – that is to nourish adequately.

| Warning Signals | **Risk Factors** | Living alone | Housebound | No regular cooked meals | Low mental test score | Clinical diagnosis of depression | Chronic Bronchitis/emphysema | Gastrectomy | Poor dentition and/or |
|---|---|---|---|---|---|---|---|---|---|
| Recent unintended weight change +/− 3 kg (7 lb) shopping, preparation. or intake<br>Lack of sunlight<br>Bereavement and/or observed depression/loneliness<br>Mental confusion affecting eating<br>High alcohol consumption<br>Multiple medications/long-term medication<br>Missed meals, snacks, fluids<br>Food wastage/rejection<br>Insufficient food stores at home<br>Lack of fruits, juices, vegetables<br>Low budget for food<br>Poor nutrition knowledge | Physical disability affecting food | | | | | | | | |

Table 4  Relevant risk factors and observed warning signals

The next group in Table 2 is people with cancer. Between episodes of chemotherapy and radiotherapy people go home, often with little or no taste sensation, with nausea and vomiting. They are a very difficult group to help, but one that really needs assistance.

Then dysphagia itself – treated separately because it needs a little more attention. There is a new approach to dysphagia now that it is possible to involve the speech therapists. Until recently, dieticians had nothing to go by other than the carer's observation of what their patients could manage. If someone appeared only to be able to manage liquid foods then that is what they were given. But now speech therapist are able to do swallowing assessments, they can give us a much clearer picture of what texture we can feed safely, and the safety of oral feeding in itself.

A disordered or absent swallow means that you can aspirate food and liquids sometimes unknowingly. This can cause choking, discomfort or pain which are frightening and may cause people to avoid eating without always saying why.

**Are there many people like this in the community?**
Well, in truth, we don't know, hence the audit into who has what problem in the community. In particular, we do not know whether all those with silent aspiration are being identified.

**Assessment of problems**
Once you have identified those with problems then a nutritional screening is necessary but that has to be evaluated in the context of the social and other factors already mentioned. If what people are saying does not seem to match up with what you are observing then it could well be worth investigating a little further. Are they telling the truth? Is that because they have not noticed they are not eating as much. If their appetite has gone down as well as their intake they will still be feeling satisfied. Is it that they do not want to be bothered? Back to the apathy again. Is it deliberate? Do they not want to lose their independence? Is it because they are denying the problem? Or are they just plain confused?

## 2 HOW AND WHAT DO WE FEED THEM?

There are three options:

Oral

Enteral (nasogastric/gastostomy)

Parenteral

I am not going to discuss Parenteral because I have no experience of Parenteral in the community. This method is properly used with in-patients.

**Oral feeding** is the method of choice if you can feed enough and feed it safely by that route. I sometimes come up against the strong feeling of people who do not use our service much. Their view seems to be 'don't let the dieticians in, they'll want to put a tube down'. But dieticians try to keep people eating normal food by the normal route for as long as possible. In addition there is the advantage of your own choice of food. It can be modified. Dieticians can supplement the food itself, making it more nutritionally dense. Remember that if you are going to puree food then the more liquid you add the more volume you get with consequent dilution. Some people end up struggling with their pureed food and getting quite full up but are really not getting very much at all. You can use all the commercial supplements but do not forget the things that can be done at home e.g. all the milky drinks which are readily available at home if there is someone to prepare them.

You can also supplement oral feeding with nasogastric or gastrostomy feeding, if people cannot take sufficient. This is particularly useful for people who have perhaps got to the stage of dribbling or being very slow with their food. Their food gets cold and they are embarrassed and they would rather not eat with the family because it really is a bit of a pain. You can often just let people eat what they want with the family (it does not matter how slow they are) if you are going to assist them perhaps with over-night or gastrostomy feeding.

There are also luncheon clubs, drop-in centres, meals on wheels: an awful lot of options open to people, providing they are available and providing they are accessible and known about by patients and carers.

Table 5 relates to modifications for people with dysphagia, not for people on soft diets simply because they are not up to a full meal. If you have an absent swallow oral feeding is just not possible. The next stage up from total non-oral feeding is to have cold semi-solid food which is a single texture and to have thickened liquids. Semi-solid is the texture of thick custard or thick yoghurt; single texture is, for example, custard without lumps i.e. one texture for your muscles to cope with at one time. Liquids are thickened because liquids are the most difficult thing to control: they tend to shoot down very quickly. If anything is going to go down the wrong way it's going to be a 'nice cup of tea'!

| | | |
|---|---|---|
| Cold semi-solid<br>Warm semi-solid | Single Texture | Thickened Liquids |
| Mixed texture<br>Soft Texture | Unthickened Liquids | |
| Normal | | |

Table 5  Non-Oral Feeding

Warm semi-solid food is slightly less well tolerated so you are improving if you get on to that. There are a number of thickeners on the market and they are improving all the time. When you get onto mixed texture you are doing quite well. The ubiquitous mince and potatoes which everyone seems to get in hospital is at least two textures: you have a gravy with little bits of mince in it and you might well have mashed potatoes and carrots which introduce a third texture.

**Enteral feeding** is on the increase in the community, partly as a result of earlier discharges from hospital. Increasingly however it is actually initiated in the community, mostly for those who are suffering from neurological disorders. This is because they do not have anything else that warrants hospital admission at that point. They are just suffering from a swallowing dysfunction.

**Can people cope with this at home?**
My experience is that people cope extremely well and have very safe and clean practices. That tends to be a self-answering question because if somebody wasn't going to cope with it very well then you would not use that system anyway.

**What do they need to cope?**

**1 Training and Support**
Firstly, if you're going to organise care in the community, there needs to be training for the patient/carer and the professional. In a hospital you tend to have a number of people in a small environment who have reasonable experience. You also need to have some support for those who are going to look after those naso-gastrically fed within the community. This is not because the community nurses are not capable or not willing but quite simply because we now have sixteen patients who are enterally fed at home whereas there were none six years ago. That means that most people do not have anyone on their case load so although we have had training days and so on, most people need someone to check things with. Also you need the authorisation ready set up so that the nurse can start the feed immediately. It is important to have district guidelines so that everyone does the same.

**2 Instructions**
Secondly the clients will need instructions in very basic language with very basic concepts particularly in infection control. We work very closely with our infection control nurses to think of things that the hospital may take for granted e.g. washing your hands and using clean surfaces.

**3 Contact numbers**
Finally you need contact numbers so that if something does go wrong somebody can be contacted quickly.

**3 FINALLY, WHAT PROBLEMS ARE THERE?**

**Care and Support**  Who is going to do all this at home? Perhaps the carers have other jobs and commitments which will interfere. Once you have decided that somebody is there to care and cook for and look after the patient, then the dietician should chat about what is required. Sometime it is all very basic and down to earth and you wonder why people have not thought about it before. However, what you are asking them to do is to change the habits of a lifetime. If someone can only manage small amounts at a time but are used to having only one main meal a day, it is surprising how often it does not occur to them to change that.

Not all carers are family or friends. With the Community Care Act we have had to extend our list of people to communicate with to the Social Services, Home Helps, Care Managers and so on. We need to have them as interested and 'onboard' as we can. If for example we have someone on cold semi-food, the last thing we need is someone to offer them a cup of hot coffee because they do not understand.

If you are going to organise meals-on-wheels you need to know whether they are available: whether there is a long waiting list. Are Drop-In Centres available to people? If you live at the top of a hill and have not got transport can you make use of the local luncheon club? Perhaps you can look to voluntary organisations. Very often they organise the local community transport rounding people up for their lunch.

An important point to be made about people who are eating normally is that there is a tendency to assume that they are eating and that there is therefore not much of a problem. Yet they are not always OK. Changes are insidious and so their nutritional status needs to be re-assessed every so often.

### Enteral feeding and getting started – Who is going to make the decision?

A lot of people must be involved in this decision, including the families of the patients and obviously the patients themselves. Families sometimes need a lot of support to come to a decision that enteral feeding is an acceptable way feeding their loved ones.

We had one lady who, like a lot of carers, was very loath to relinquish some of her burden. It was very difficult for her. The more she was encouraged that her relative was not swallowing anything, no matter how long she sat and fed him, the more she felt she was opting out of looking after him by choosing some hi-tech soulless way of feeding him. That is understandable. She agreed in the end to try enteral feeding for a very short period of time. (There is no reason to assume that nasogastric feeding is an end stage method of feeding. It can be stopped and you can go back to some other method.) She found that the time spent encouraging her relative to eat had been upsetting. With enteral feeding she spent some of that time reading the newspaper to him, which she felt was a very worthwhile exercise. So she was getting something positive out of it as well as him.

### Making the decision
Is the decision made early enough to organise everything before discharge? Long before discharge there needs to be an agreement as to who does what, who will pay. The cost of the feed comes off FP 10, the cost of the plastics is about £100 a month. It does not matter who pays as long as the budget is allocated. However, usually these costs have just crept into budgets and Purchasers need to be made aware that this is an area of changing clinical practices which in most areas is not being funded. The decision as to who pays is something which needs to be examined locally.

### How is the feed to be delivered?
Are people going to have to go down to the chemists and pick up bags and bottles or can you find a local chemist who will deliver? There are companies who will deliver to the home, but that takes time to set up. Prescriptions for the feeds as well as requests for the plastics, pumps etc. are sent off to the company. If there is advance notice that the patient is to be discharged, all should go smoothly, because the system swings into action. Unfortunately, problems may occur when people are discharged to residential homes because when a place becomes available they need to move quickly. No-one wants to keep the patient in because they are blocking beds, but if they are moving away from their normal GP a new one has to be contacted, prescriptions have to be sorted out which takes time. Once it is working it works very well but there is a time lag in getting everything sorted out.

### What do we need to do? What is needed?
Training, education and support – there needs to be a lot of communication, both multi-disciplinary and multi-agency. Guidelines and systems need to be set up so that people can just slot in.

**Awareness** – if people are not aware of the problems lack of nutrition can cause them they will not put a lot of effort into feeding. To avoid the downward spiral you must intervene as soon as possible. Not only does the spiral lead to malnutrition representing a deteriorating quality of life but also in terms of resources it would be more sensible to intervene earlier and prevent ourselves spending a lot of time, money and effort in retrieving a situation which shouldn't really have got out of hand in the first place.

### ADDRESS FOR CORRESPONDENCE

Miss E Oliver
Manager, Nutrition and Dietetics
Milton Keynes General Hospital,
Standing Way,
Eaglestone,
Milton Keynes
MK6 5LD

## QUESTIONS TO CONSIDER WHEN SELECTING EQUIPMENT[13]

■ What is the patient's risk of pressure sore development? Patients in high-risk categories usually require more sophisticated equipment.

■ Has the patient existing pressure damage and, if so, how severe is it? Patients with pressure sores are likely to need a pressure-relieving mattress or one of the more sophisticated pressure-reducing systems.

■ How many hours each day does the patient spend in bed? If a patient spends long periods in bed, effective pressure relief/reduction is essential.

■ Can the patient move unaided? If so, simple static systems may be effective.

■ Is the patient starting to rehabilitate, for example, getting in and out of bed. The support system should not raise the bed too high, and the bed should be easy for the patient to move on and have a firm edge.

■ Is the patient difficult to move or can he/she lie in only one position? A bed with electric controls such as a low-air-loss bed may be most appropriate.

■ What are the main objectives of treatment? For example, is the patient terminally ill and in pain when being moved? In this situation a sophisticated system that reduces the frequency required for repositioning the patient would be appropriate.

■ What is the patient's weight? Is the patient too heavy/light for the chosen equipment?

# PRESSURE-RELIEVING/ REDUCING MATTRESSES

Carol Dealey, BSc(Hons), RGN, RCNT, is clinical nurse specialist in tissue viability, Community Hospitals Division, Southern Birmingham Community Health NHS Trust

## EXAMPLES OF MATTRESSES AND BEDS

**Air support systems**
■ Alternating air overlays – Alpha X-Cell, Biwave, PPS 1000
■ Alternating air mattresses – Astec, Autoxcell, Biwave Plus, PPS 2000, Quatro
■ Static air flotation overlays – Airtech Topper, Roho, Waffle Floatation System
■ Low-air-loss overlays – Alamo, Clinirest, Paragon Convertible
■ Low-air-loss mattresses – Biomed X, OSA 1000, Paragon
■ Low-air-loss beds – Acucare, BioDyne II, Kinair III, Low Flow Therapy, Mediscus Monarch, Paragon 3500, Therapulse
■ Air fluidised beds – Clinitron, FluidAir Plus, Paragon 5000
■ Dynamic air flotation mattress – Nimbus,
■ Airwave mattress – Pegasus

**Fibre and foam support systems**
■ Fibre systems – Bodypillo, Charnwood Comfort, Hygiarelief, Permaflow, Permalux, Snuggledown, Spenco, Superdown, Surgic goods, Transoft
■ Foam support overlays – Modular Pro Pad, Pressure Guard
■ Foam support mattresses – Omnifoam Plus, Preventix, Softfoam, Transfoam, Vaperm

**Gel support systems**
■ Gel overlays – Action Pads, Tendercare
■ Gel mattress – Charnwood LDC

**Water support systems**
■ Water overlays – Ardo, Elwa
■ Water beds – Beaufort-Winchester, Guardian 1250

## PRESSURE-RELIEVING MATTRESS

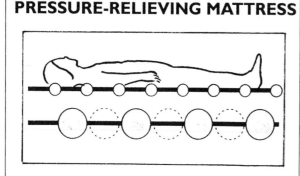

A mattress which moves in a cyclical manner, subjecting alternating areas of the body to low pressures, allowing reperfusion of tissues and pressure sore prevention.

## PRESSURE-REDUCING MATTRESS

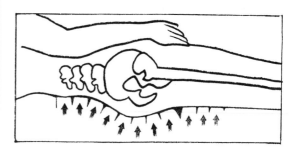

This type of mattress moulds around the body, increasing the area in contact with support. The load is more widely distributed and pressure reduced at bony prominences.

## GLOSSARY OF TERMS

■ Support system: A term which describes all types of pressure-relieving/reducing equipment.

■ Overlay mattress: A support system which is placed on top of an ordinary mattress.

■ Bed: A system comprising an integral bed frame and mattress

■ Dynamic system: A support system which alters pressure during use, for example, those with inflating and deflating cells.

■ Static system: A support system which does not alter once it has been set up. Pressure is reduced by spreading weight over a large area.

## FLOW CHART FOR SELECTING MATTRESSES*

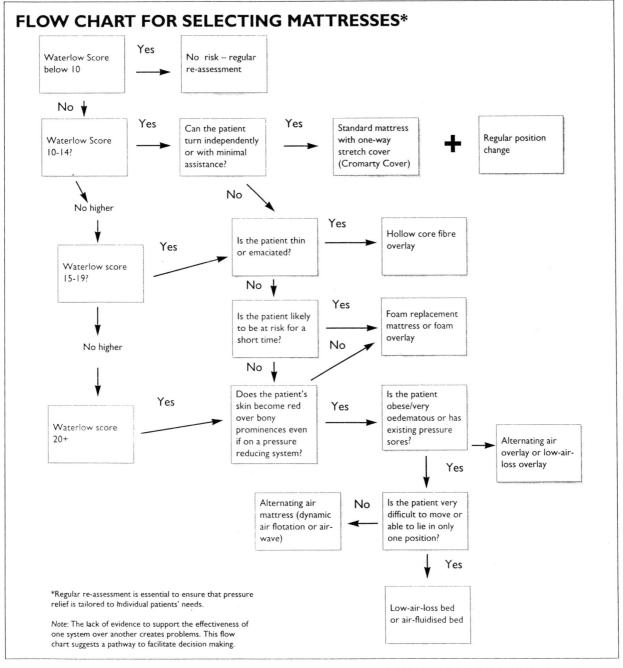

*Regular re-assessment is essential to ensure that pressure relief is tailored to individual patients' needs.

Note: The lack of evidence to support the effectiveness of one system over another creates problems. This flow chart suggests a pathway to facilitate decision making.

POSITIONING

# POSITIONING for COMFORT and PRESSURE RELIEF

Positioning for comfort and effective pressure relief is achievable using any one of a wide range of commercially available support systems, or by careful positioning using soft pillows, foam wedges and/or bead pillows, etc.

As the illustrations below show, the underlying principle is to distribute support and pressure as widely as possible by *'spreading the load'* and eliminating localised areas of high pressure. Provided this principle is followed, comfort and effective pressure relief can be achieved even in the most awkward and unusual situations.

1

*Note the areas which are not supported entirely.*

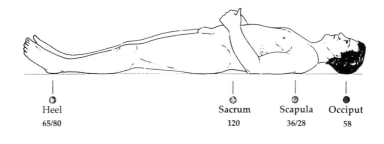

| Heel | Sacrum | Scapula | Occiput |
|------|--------|---------|---------|
| 65/80 | 120 | 36/28 | 58 |

Pressure values, experienced by a male subject of average build, weight 12½ stone, lying on a hard surface, were as shown. (Values expressed in mm/Hg obtained using Talley Scimedics Skin Pressure Evaluator MK III).

Remember the maxim *'if there's a space – fill it!'* and provide cushioning of sufficient depth to provide support without excessive disruption of the natural body contours and alignment. How effective applying this principle can be is illustrated below.
*N.B. Small pieces of sheepskin/fleece can be particularly useful for supporting small areas.*

# P O S I T I O N

2

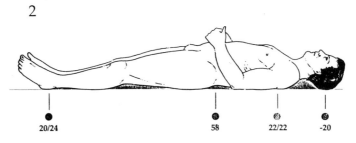

| 20/24 | 58 | 22/22 | -20 |
|-------|-----|-------|-----|

Tolerance of *'hard'* sites to pressure is low. Whenever possible, patients should be positioned so that pressure is shifted to more tolerant *'soft'* sites (buttocks, thighs etc.).

The 30 degree tilt technique is particularly effective at this and is most useful for bedridden patients. The illustrations on the following pages demonstrate the basic procedure, but provided the principle described above is adhered to, many other variants of positioning may be followed with much greater comfort, safety and ease of practice for both patient and operator.

The same subject with cushioning in lumbar, popliteal and Achilles tendon spaces, showing the reduction in pressure over the sites measured.

*In circumstances where recumbent positioning on hard surfaces is unavoidable, the above practice is the absolute minimum to help prevent/limit pressure damage.*

## RECUMBENT POSITIONING

No one positioning technique is suitable for the wide range of conditions and situations encountered in general nursing practice. The principle of 'spreading the load' will, however, if followed, do much to greatly improve the comfort and resistance to pressure damage of the majority of patients. Illustrations are given of three example positions and how to achieve them – it is hoped these will provide pointers for application in other situations.

For many bedridden patients the basic 30 degree tilt position will be found most suitable in either its recumbent or semi-recumbent forms.

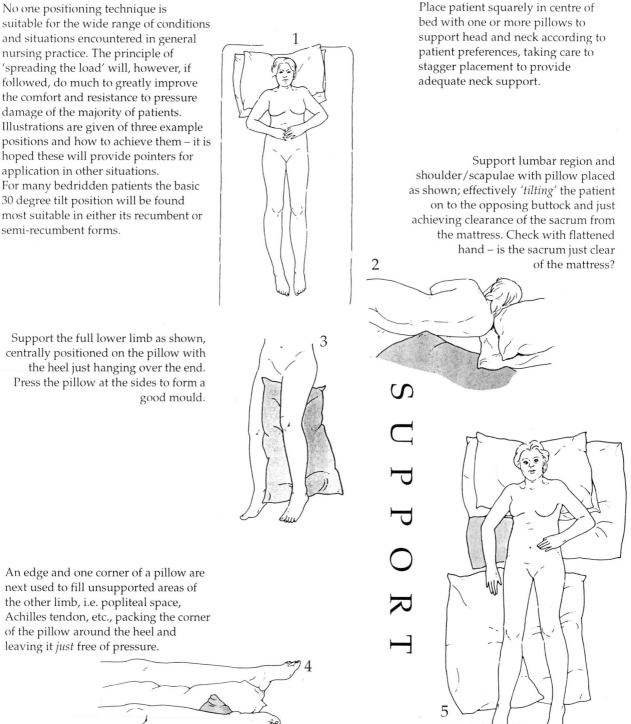

Place patient squarely in centre of bed with one or more pillows to support head and neck according to patient preferences, taking care to stagger placement to provide adequate neck support.

Support lumbar region and shoulder/scapulae with pillow placed as shown; effectively *'tilting'* the patient on to the opposing buttock and just achieving clearance of the sacrum from the mattress. Check with flattened hand – is the sacrum just clear of the mattress?

Support the full lower limb as shown, centrally positioned on the pillow with the heel just hanging over the end. Press the pillow at the sides to form a good mould.

An edge and one corner of a pillow are next used to fill unsupported areas of the other limb, i.e. popliteal space, Achilles tendon, etc., packing the corner of the pillow around the heel and leaving it *just* free of pressure.

S U P P O R T

For extra comfort the use of another pillow, cushion or even rolled up blanket to support the right arm and shoulder may be found helpful.

## SEMI-RECUMBENT POSITIONING

Forward slide is the most frequent complication of this form of positioning giving rise to damaging friction and shearing forces.

Raising the foot of the bed by about three inches will provide a counter force and greatly limit forward slide. In normal practice it may be found possible to leave most hospital beds with this amount of tilt as standard.

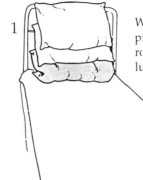

1

With the back rest out place three pillows as shown with the lower one rolled or *'plumped up'* to provide good lumbar support.

C O M F O R T

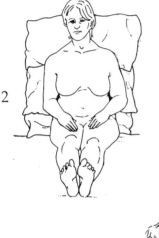

2

Place the patient firmly up against the pillows ensuring that he/she is *lifted clear* of the bottom sheets to avoid friction and skin damage.

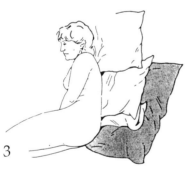

3

With the patient's buttock lifted clear of the bed a pillow *corner only* is placed under the buttock to *'tilt'* the body and give clearance to ischium and sacrum. The rest of the pillow is placed under the other pillows as shown to give greater support for the back.

*N.B. If feather pillows are being used ensure that the corner has sufficient filling by 'shaking down' the pillow.*

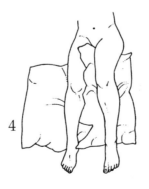

4

The lower limbs are now supported as before just ensuring heel clearance from the mattress.

Finally position another pillow under those against the back rest to support the other side and give greater comfort and security for the patient.

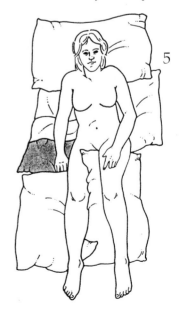

5

## VARIANT POSITIONS

Some patients pose particular difficulties because of problems such as contractures of limbs or their poor mental state. In such cases positioning options may be very limited. In these situations it is important to follow the basic principle of providing maximum support and ensure that all vulnerable sites are protected.

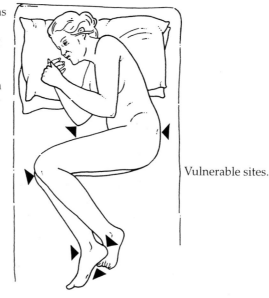

Vulnerable sites.

1

# S T A B I L I T Y

In this illustration pillows have been positioned as shown and the most vulnerable sites almost completely protected with the patient much more comfortable and relaxed because of the support. The use of Tubipads or similar will help to protect elbows but these should seldom be necessary for heels if the technique is followed correctly.

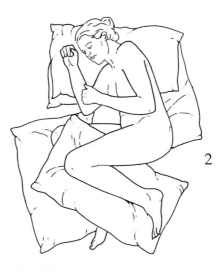

2

*Where situations such as this are encountered it is strongly advisable to use a specialist support system in conjunction with the above measures if at all possible.*

Reference and Further Reading;

*Preston K W - Positioning for Comfort and Pressure Relief: The 30 Degree Alternative. CARE – Science and Practice, Vol. 6, no. 4, December 1988, 116–119.*

*Seiler W O, Allen S, Stahelin H B (1986) – Influence of the 30 degree laterally inclined position and the 'Supersoft' 3 piece mattress on skin oxygen tension on areas of maximum pressure - implication for Pressure Sore Prevention; Gerontology 32:158–166.*

*Seiler W O, Stahelin H B (1979) – Skin oxygen tension as a function of imposed skin pressure – implication for decubitus ulcer formation; J of Am Geriatric Society; Vol XXVII, 7, 298–301.*

And for theatre areas; *Anderton J M, Keen R I, Neave R – Positioning the Surgical Patient. Butterworth (1988) ISBN - 407 01220-6.*

*Limitations on space have prevented consideration of the needs of chair bound patients in this paper. It is hoped to produce a further chart, illustrating methods of positioning for comfort and pressure relief for such patients in the near future.*

Illustrations by Jonathan Boat
Designed by Lorraine Clark
Lincolnshire College of Art and Design.

Acknowledgement; The support of CONVATEC, makers of GRANUFLEX, with the production of this chart is gratefully acknowledged.

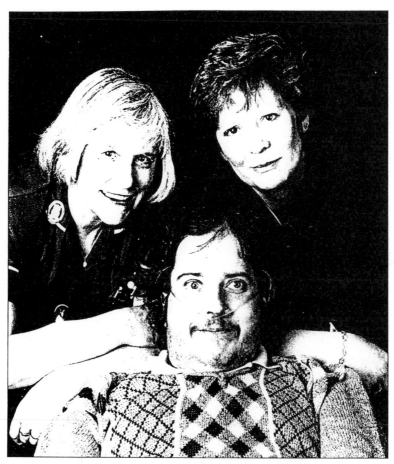

Val Evans (left), district nurse, and Mair Fear, research nurse,
with John: an effective team approach

# JOHN'S STORY

One patient was greatly helped by a community nurse and a research nurse

working together as a team and by the appropriate selection of dressings.

Val Evans, Mair Fear and the patient, John, each give their perspective

My name is John. I am 26 years old and I would like to tell you about a pressure sore I have and how it affects me.

The biggest problem is that it has kept me in hospital for long periods, and I hate being in hospital. As soon as I go through the doors I feel miserable. One of the worst things is the boredom. All I can do is read or watch television, and I soon get tired of that. The nurses are pleasant, but as I am not the only person they have to look after they can only spend so much time with me. The highlight of my day is when my wife and friends come to see me. This isn't always easy, as they have to arrange transport which can become expensive. I dread seeing my wife leave. All I want is to be with her at home.

Over the years, I have spend long periods in hospital; the longest was when I had a pressure sore grafted and the graft didn't take. That is what I was afraid might happen on this last occasion. When the research nurse came to see me I thought: Here comes another one to look at my bottom! She showed me a tracing of the pressure sore and this was the first time I realised what it looked like. After talking to me for a long time she said that she was going to try a new dressing and, provided I did my lifting exercises regularly to relieve the pressure on the area and allow the blood to circulate properly, it might help improve my condition. Although I had been told previously that these exercises were important, I hadn't really understood why.

Now I am home again, and when the nurses come to see me they show me new tracings and photographs of my sore and discuss the improvement with me. Although I am not always familiar with the terms they use, I am beginning to understand them and it is good to see the nurses looking pleased with my progress. The new dressing doesn't need changing as often as the others, so that gives my wife and I more time to spend together. I have a nice home and my wife looks after it and me very well. That's all I want.

## THE COMMUNITY NURSE'S VIEW

John was transferred into our care in July 1991. He has spina bifida and as a result is paraplegic and confined to a wheelchair. His urinary continence is managed with an indwelling catheter. For the past seven years he has also suffered from epilepsy, but this is well controlled with medication. Hodgkin's disease was diagnosed in 1991 and, although John received some chemotherapy, he was unable to tolerate it and therefore could not complete the treatment. His pain is controlled with subcutaneous diamorphine via a syringe driver. Despite his poor medical condition John is a cheerful and well-adjusted man with a terrific sense of humour.

A nursing assessment of John's physical, social and psychological condition was carried out so that a suitable care plan could be devised.

It appeared that his pressure sore caused him most distress, not through pain (he cannot feel it) but because of the associated inconvenience. He has previously been admitted to hospital for skin grafting, and the possibility of further hospital admission also caused him concern.

His other problems, in order of importance to him, were identified as the epilepsy, which he wanted to keep well controlled; the catheter, which sometimes leaked and which had caused some necrosis to the urethral orifice of the glans penis; the syringe driver, because it required frequent nursing attention; and the Hodgkin's disease, which he knew was progressive.

John did not see as a major problem the spina bifida and maintenance of his Spitz Holtzer valve. When first examined, his pressure sore, which involved a large part of the sacral and gluteal regions, was found to be relatively clean and healthy in appearance and therefore the existing treatment was continued. This consisted of packing the wound twice daily with alginate dressings, with Gamgee tissue applied to absorb any excess exudate. After a couple of weeks, dressing changes were reduced to once a day and closely monitored, as evening visits were restricting both John's family and social life. Bowel movements did not generally cause contamination of the wound as they were relatively regular, occurring early in the morning well before the arrival of the district nurse who could instigate dressing changes if soiling had occurred.

In October 1991 John was admitted to the local general hospital with a urinary infection and an abscess in the lymph vessels in his groin. He also developed an infection in his pressure sore and was referred to the research nurse for advice and recommendations for the treatment of this area.

Since his discharge John's wound has improved considerably. The new dressings are easy to use and do not crumple or become lumpy like Gamgee tissue. Changes are easily accomplished and these have recently been reduced to every third day unless leakage from the catheter necessitates a more frequent change. The improvement has encouraged John to persevere with the pressure-relieving exercises and these, in turn, have assisted in the healing process.

## THE RESEARCH NURSE'S VIEW

John was first seen in the ward following a request from hospital staff for advice on the treatment of his pressure sore. This was a large area which included a bridge of tissue over a heavily exuding cavity coated with slough. His diagnosis and prognosis were such that it was not considered likely that his wound would heal very rapidly, but his paraplegia meant that it did not cause him any pain or discomfort. He therefore viewed the problem primarily as a hindrance to his family and social life, as before his admission dressing regimes sometimes required changing twice or even three times a day. This meant that he was tied to the home and deprived of the privacy and independence he desired.

John was very unhappy in hospital and his anxieties were compounded by the fact that he had been told that he would not be discharged until a special pressure-relieving bed could be obtained for his home. John had been married only six months and was living with his wife in a small flat within a complex for handicapped people. There was one bed in the flat which they shared. The introduction of a different bed would mean that he and his wife would have to sleep apart — a situation he found unacceptable.

The nature and characteristics of the wound were such that before John could be discharged from hospital a dressing regimen was required which met the following criteria:

■ The dressing for the cavity should possess significant bulk and conform to the contours of the wound

■ It should be able to absorb significant amounts of exudate and not require changing more than once a day — less frequently if possible

■ For the area around the cavity the dressing should also be absorbent and not adhere to the surface of the wound or cause maceration of the surrounding skin

■ The materials chosen should not apply further pressure to the wound, as John would be spending quite long periods of time in a sitting position

■ The method of retention should be comfortable and conforming in order to maintain the dressings for long periods without producing the skin damage that had occurred with tapes used previously.

Allevyn cavity wound dressing and Allevyn foam sheet were selected, because the foam used in the manufacture of both dressings is soft and resilient and laboratory studies have shown that it is capable of absorbing and retaining large volumes of fluid even under pressure.[1] In addition, experience has shown that the Allevyn sheet dressing is unlikely to adhere to the surface of the wound and cause trauma upon removal. Both dressings are also easy to apply and remove and do not require John to spend long periods of time in positions that he finds uncomfortable.

It was emphasised to John that he should ensure that his diet was adequate and that it should include sufficient protein, zinc, vitamin C and carbohydrate to promote healing.[2-4] He also had to remain well hydrated and drink at least two litres of fluid daily to help catheter drainage. John also agreed to lift himself off his buttocks at regular intervals, at least once every two hours.

**John's dressings are easy to use and changes are easily accomplished**

Once John's infection was brought under control, the medical and nursing staff in the ward agreed to his discharge. The research nurse met with district nursing staff responsible for John's care to discuss the new treatment, the first of a series of regular meetings in which John's progress was reviewed and discussed.

## THE OUTCOME

Once John had been discharged, district nurses visited him each morning to help get him out of bed and perform dressing changes as required. Although John experienced problems with his catheter and was awaiting a suprapubic one, wound healing had not been inhibited, but dressing changes took place more frequently than would otherwise have been the case. John continued to take an active interest in the tracings of his wound which confirmed that healing was taking place, and he looked forward to a time when dressing changes would not be required.

Because Allevyn dressings are not available on prescription, supplies had to be obtained via the research nurse. In 33 days, 17 dressing changes were performed, 12 of which were for routine inspection. The dressings generally remained undisturbed for two days and changes were often required only because of catheter leakage. Although the

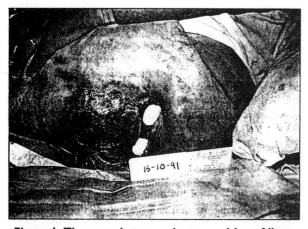

**Figure 1. The wound at an early stage, with an Allevyn cavity wound dressing clearly visible under the bridge of tissue**

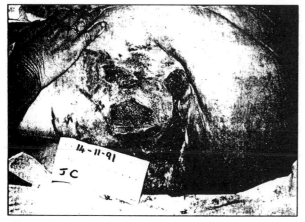

**Figure 2. The wound four weeks later showing obvious signs of improvement**

dressings are relatively expensive on a unit cost basis, they can be extremely cost-effective, as in this instance; a major improvement in the wound was noted and signs of healing were evident (Figures 1 and 2).

John's case confirmed once again that the range of products available to district nurses is not always adequate to allow them to provide the best treatment for their patients.[5,6] Products are often too small or insufficiently absorbent to cope with the exudate or they may be unable to contain an offensive odour that can permeate through wads of Gamgee tissue.

When prescribing wound care, emphasis is generally directed to an accurate assessment of the wound size, condition and location, together with other factors that may influence the healing process,[7-10] but patients' individual needs and requirements are not always considered.[11]

John was an outgoing and extrovert person who had no intention of spending 24 hours confined to his flat, let alone his bed. John and his wife enjoyed the time they spent together and were fortunate to have the support of their friends. They received regular visits from members of the primary health care team whom they could contact by telephone at any time.

In this instance, the team approach to the management of John's pressure sore worked well, with John playing an active rather than passive role in his own care. This illustrates the importance of the need for professionals to work together with their patients or clients to ensure cooperation and understanding of each other's problems. It also emphasises that it is the role of the specialist nurse to act as a resource[12] and not to seek to erode the vital role played by the community nursing staff. ■

■ Since this article was written, John has had to spend a further period in hospital because of his Hodgkin's disease and problems with his suprapubic catheter. The district nurse is attempting to obtain an electric wheelchair for him to use when he returns home, as he finds his manual one a little difficult to manoeuvre in the disco!

REFERENCES
[1] Thomas, S. *Wound Management and Dressings.* London: Pharmaceutical Press, 1991.
[2] Hanan, K., Scheele, L., Albumen weight as a predictor of nutritional status and pressure ulcer development. *Ostomy/Wound Management* 1991; **33**: 22–27.
[3] Millar, B., Torrance, C. Nutritional assessment. *Surgical Nurse* 1991; **4**: 5, 21–26.
[4] Brown, K. The role of nutrition in pressure area care. *Journal of Tissue Viability* 1991; **13**: 63–64.
[5] Bale, S. A dilemma in the community. *Nursing Standard* 1988; **2**: 30, 33–34.
[6] Milward, P, Practical problems of wound care in the community. *Wound Management* 1991; **1**: 3, 6–8.
[7] Morrison, J.M. Pressure sores: assessing the wound. *Professional Nurse* 1989; **4**: 5, 32–535.
[8] Dobrzanski, S. Furness, S., Lister, J. Pressure sore documents. *Journal of Tissue Viability* 1991; **1**: 4, 99–102.
[9] Dealey, C. Assessing wounds and selecting dressings. *Nursing Standard* (Society for Tissue Viability Supplement ) 1990; **7**: 8–10.
[10] Thomas, S. Selecting dressings. *Community Outlook* 1991; **1**: 6, 28–33
[11] Poulton, B. Factors which influence patient compliance. *Journal of Tissue Viability* 1991; **1**: 4, 108–110
[12] Dealey, C. The role of the tissue viability nurse. *Nursing Standard* (Society for Tissue Viability Supplement) 1988; **2**: 4–5

Val Evans, RGN, RMNS, NDN, is a district nurse, Taff Ely/Rhondda. Mair Fear, RGN, NDN Cert, is research nurse, tissue viability, Surgical Materials Testing Laboratory, Bridgend General Hospital, Mid Glamorgan

# Development of the link-nurse role in clinical settings

**KEY WORDS**

Networking, clinical nurse
specialists

**ABSTRACT**

The link-nurse scheme appears to
be one way of narrowing the gap
between theory and practice. This
paper examines the concept, role,
history and evolution of link nurses
and, based on the author's personal
experience of direct involvement in
such a scheme, attempts to identify
some of its advantages and
drawbacks

*Liz Charalambous, RGN,
primary nurse, care of older
people, University Hospital,
Queen's Medical Centre,
Nottingham*

NURSING ROLES HAVE undergone many recent changes, including primary nursing and those changes that came about because of the introduction of clinical grading. This has resulted in nurses who are ambitious for higher grades being invariably discouraged from changing from clinical areas, which means greater specialisation at an early stage in their careers.

Although qualified nurses have a responsibility to update their practice,[1] this can be difficult because of constraints on time and the speed with which theory and practice change. It would be impossible for a specialist nurse to assess and plan the care of individual patients along with the other responsibilities of being staff advocate, practitioner, educator, consultant, researcher and change agent.[2]

It has also been suggested that in order to meet the health needs of a nation, the nursing profession needs scholarly practitioners who can translate their advanced preparation into practice.[3]

So how can clinically based nurses provide a good standard of care? To solve this problem, many hospitals are organising a network of link-nurse schemes in which the senior nurse for a clinical specialty invites a nurse from each ward to become a link person between the clinical nurse specialist and his or her ward. The role involves attendance at meetings where ideas and new developments can be discussed and feeding back the relevant information to nurses in the ward which, in turn, can help communication with patients and their families (Fig 1). Ching's experience demonstrates how infection control link nurses can help to motivate ward staff to comply with any control measures that are introduced.[4]

The main clinical specialties include nutrition, infection control, continence, swallowing and wound care. However, the possibilities are endless; diabetes, care of older people, paediatric, respiratory, HIV and teaching are just a few examples of areas needing attention.

A review of the literature reveals that little has been written on the subject. The term clinical nurse specialist began to appear in the mid 1960s[5] and by the late 1960s and early 1970s it became accepted that advancement within the profession should not always necessitate a move away from the bedside.[6] The idea that nurses should consult other nurses outside their immediate work group was a relatively new concept in

the 1980s.[7,8] In 1983, Fife and Lemler suggested that one way clinical nurse specialists could use their roles as educators was through conversations with nurses about existing problems and needs.[9] Fenton describes how the clinical nurse specialist could use formal and informal contacts to work around bureaucratic blocks to benefit the patient.[10]

Hospitals need link nurses to act as vital bridges between theory and practice. Storr suggests that one way to bridge the gap between theory and practice is through active utilisation of the clinical nurse specialist position.[2] The Dreyfus model[11] suggests that the theoretician must always depend on the practitioner for clinical knowledge development and for finding questions that current theorising does not cover. Likewise, the clinical nurse specialist depends on the link nurse to raise questions relating to the care needs of patients in his or her specialty. Conversely, the link nurse at ward level relies on the clinical nurse specialist to supply her with accurate, relevant and up-to-date information.

Skills based on experience are not always easy to grasp conceptually. The beginner must operate on abstract principles, formal models and theories in order to learn safely and efficiently. However, with experience, the clinical nurse specialist develops knowledge from which to make rapid clinical decisions and judgements based on concrete examples.[12] Thus, a symbiotic relationship emerges between the clinical nurse specialist and link nurse. Ching found that link schemes improved the quality of patient care and raised nurses' awareness of clinical issues.[4]

A minimum background knowledge is required to be a good link nurse and also the ability to pass on information and be in a position to implement change at ward level, so for these reasons only registered nurses may attend. The ideal link nurse should be a keen, enthusiastic, motivated volunteer, who has a special interest in a particular specialty. Good teaching and presentation skills are necessary, as is a charismatic approach in order to encourage colleagues to practise up-to-date, research-based skills. Gibson outlines how enthusiasm and organisation made the link-nurse team for continence a success in her area.[13] Nottingham nutritional link nurses devised and then implemented an assessment tool to detect patients at risk from malnutrition.[14]

**Box 1. Potential drawbacks of the link-nurse scheme**

The financial incentives of the reformed NHS mean managers place a greater emphasis on value for money, which means the hours of nursing time spent away from patient care attending link nurse meetings must be accounted for. Managers have the added problem (and cost) of evaluating the effectiveness of the link-nurse scheme.

Second, clinical nurse specialists may feel fearful of having their role eroded because of the increasing expertise of their link nurses.

Third, nurses may have problems attending the meetings owing to clinical pressures, unforeseen workload, night duty rotation and holidays. New link nurses may feel at a disadvantage if they join well-established groups. However, feelings of insecurity can be eliminated by the clinical nurse specialist offering support.[15] This should be supplemented by comprehensive written information describing the role profile, philosophy and aims and objectives of the scheme.

The implications of these hidden costs are realised only when a link nurse leaves the clinical area and a replacement has to be found. Link-nurse schemes currently offer no financial incentives or evidence of study such as a formal qualification (although the ENB has started looking at this). The added value of the role to a nurse's career development is difficult to justify, as there are no national standards. For this reason it may be necessary to consider validating the role as part of PREP requirements.

It has to be acknowledged that schemes may provide a readily available escape from the pressure of ward work, with few benefits to the patient and ward team. Nurses may be fearful of admitting to a lack of knowledge or existing bad practice to the clinical nurse specialist.[17] Nurses also need to question whether the patient is in danger of becoming smothered by protocols and red tape and whether we are in danger of losing confidence in our judgements. We must beware of fitting the patient around the care rather than fitting the care around the patient

**Fig 1. The communications role of the link nurse**

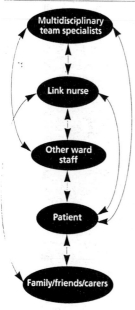

Problems may occur if members of staff are forced to attend meetings about something in which they have no particular interest or if they come from a clinical area that is resistant to change (see Box 1). The clinical nurse specialist also needs to be approachable and, to some extent, readily available; ward managers need to take account of link-nurse meetings and make allowances for staff participating in the scheme by effective off-duty planning.

The benefit of the link-nurse scheme is that communication between ward nurses and specialist nurses has the potential to improve, which can lead to an increase in the quality of care provided to the patient. The link-nurse scheme appears to have narrowed the gap between theory and practice, and there is evidence to suggest that clinical practice has improved as a direct result.[4]

There are also interesting possibilities; for example, in the field of infection control, Horton outlined to the ENB a course curriculum designed to 'produce a practitioner who is able to create and maintain an environment that will ensure the safety of the patient, his relatives and health care workers, using infection control knowledge, nursing skills and attitudes appropriate to each situation'.[15]

They devised a role profile for the link nurse aimed at enabling him or her to understand the rationale behind actions and to provide the confidence to discuss or argue a point when faced with opposition. Another possibility is that, if properly trained, link nurses can be involved in auditing and the collection of data.[16]

Link nurses can feed back information by presenting a display or keeping a folder in the ward, which should be accessible, especially if they are off duty. Some use an informal discussion format, while others prefer a more formal approach such as a teaching session. As link nurses become more fluent in their new nursing skills and knowledge they will set an example by their actions and this will improve the quality of care.

Finally, in the rush to develop links between theory and practice there is a risk that the link nurse may become a faded replica of the specialist. There is an inherent danger that the knowledge and skills invested in the ward nurse may become another referral point for the patient who may have to wait several days for an assessment.

It is only through the sharing of knowledge and the dissemination of information throughout the team that the patient will experience timely, effective and research-based care.

The idea of the link-nurse scheme appears to be taking off and as a result there is evidence of a closer liaison between theory and practice. However, it is clear from the literature that further research into the effectiveness of the link nurse in raising the standard of patient care is needed. **NT**

REFERENCES
[1]UKCC. *Professional Code of Conduct.* London: UKCC, 1992.
[2]Storr, G. The clinical nurse specialist: from the outside looking in. *Journal of Advanced Nursing* 1988; **13**: 265–272.
[3]Dirschel, K.M. The conception, gestation and delivery of the clinical nursing specialist. In: Rotkovitch, R. (ed). *Quality Patient Care and the Role of the Clinical Nursing Specialist.* New York: John Wiley, 1976.
[4]Ching, T.Y. Evaluating the efficacy of the infection control liaison nurse in one hospital. *Journal of Advanced Nursing* 1990; **15**: 1128–1131.
[5]Hamric, A. Role development and functions. In: Hamric, A.B., Spross, J. (eds). *The Clinical Nurse Specialist in Theory and Practice.* New York: Grune and Stratton, 1983.
[6]Mallison, M. The shoes of the clinician. *The American Journal of Nursing* 1984; **84**: 587.
[7]Barron, A. The CNS as consultant. In: Hamrick, A.B., Spross, J. (eds). *The Clinical Nurse Specialist in Theory and Practice.* New York: Grune and Stratton, 1983.
[8]Everson, S. Integration of the role of the clinical nurse specialist. *Journal of Continuing Education in Nursing* 1982; **12**: 2, 16–19.
[9]Fife, B., Lemler, S. The psychiatric nurse specialist: a valuable asset in the general hospital. *Journal of Nursing Administration* 1983; **13**: 4, 14–17.
[10]Fenton, M. Identifying competencies of clinical nurse specialists. *Journal of Nursing Administration* 1985; **15**: 12, 31–37.
[11]Dreyfus, S.E., Dreyfus, H.L. *A Five-Stage Model of the Mental Activities Involved in Directed Skill Acquisition* (unpublished report). Berkeley, Ca.: University of California, 1980.
[12]Benner, P. *From Novice to Expert: Excellence and Power in Clinical Nursing Practice.* Menlo Park, Ca.: Addison-Wesley Publishing, 1984.
[13]Gibson, E. Coordinating continence care. *Nursing Times* 1989; **85**: 7, 75.
[14]Charalambous, L. A healthy approach. *Nursing Times* 1993; **89**: 20, 58–60.
[15]Horton, R. Linking the chain. *Nursing Times* 1988; **84**: 26, 44–46.
[16]Dearden, D. *Developing an Infection Control Link-Nurse Network at University Hospital, Nottingham* (unpublished dissertation). Nottingham: Trent University, 1993.
[17]Edlund, B., Hodges, L. Preparing and using the clinical nurse specialist. *Nursing Ethics of North America* 1983; **18**: 499–507.

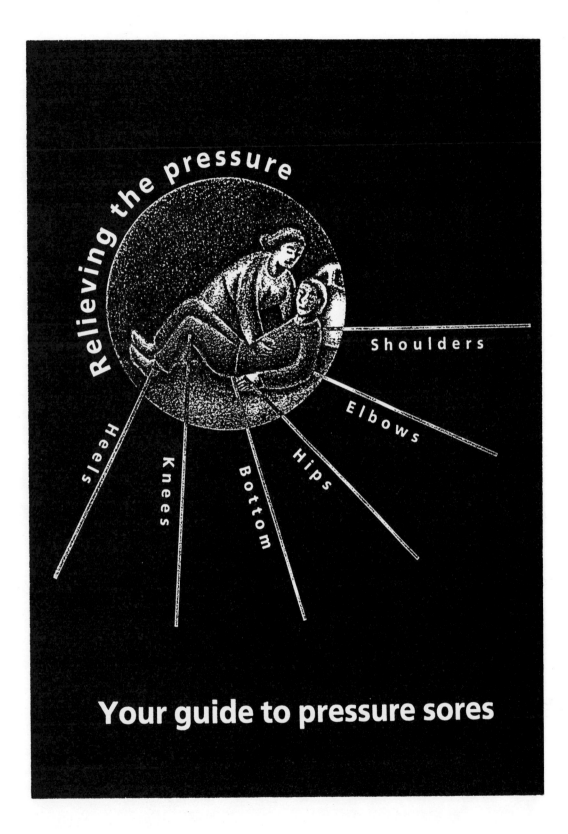

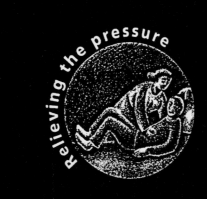

Relieving the pressure

If you have to stay in bed or if you spend most of your time in a wheelchair or armchair, the last thing you need is a pressure sore. These painful wounds are sometimes known as 'bedsores', and they can take months to heal. If they become infected they can even kill.

**Carers** If you are looking after someone who has to spend time in a bed, chair or wheelchair, you should find this booklet useful. There are extra notes in boxes like this to help you.

## ❓ What is a pressure sore?

A pressure sore is an area of damaged skin and flesh. It is usually caused by sitting or lying in one position for too long without moving.

A pressure sore can develop in only a few hours. It usually starts with the skin changing colour – it may appear slightly redder or darker than usual. If a sore isn't treated quickly, it can develop in a few days into an open blister and – over a longer period – into a deep hole in the flesh.

Sores are most likely to develop on the parts of the body which take your weight and where the bone is close to the surface. The areas most at risk are the heels, ankles, knees, hips, bottom, base of the spine, elbows and shoulders.

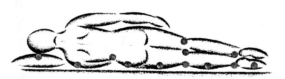

## ❓ Who is most likely to get a pressure sore?

You are more likely to get a pressure sore if:

- you have to stay in bed
- you are in a wheelchair
- you spend long periods in an armchair
- you have difficulty moving about
- you are elderly or weak
- you have a serious illness
- you are incontinent
- your body is not very sensitive, for example because you are diabetic or have had a stroke
- you have a bad heart or poor circulation
- you are not eating a balanced diet or having enough to drink

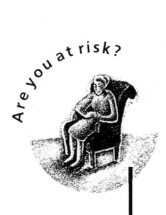

Are you at risk?

**You don't have to be stuck in bed to get a pressure sore**

---

**Carers**

- People who cannot change position without help are at great risk.
- People who are less mentally aware (for example, because of Alzheimer's disease or heavy sedation) are also at risk.

How can I avoid pressure sores?

Prevention is much better than cure. The best way to avoid getting a sore is to get out of your bed or chair for a short walk every hour or so. This gets the blood flowing and helps tone up the muscles. But not everyone can manage this, and there are other ways to avoid pressure sores.

**If you are in bed:**

**The best way to avoid getting a sore is to get moving**

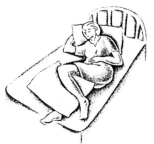

- If possible, change your position at least every two hours, alternating between your back and your sides. You may need help to do this properly so that you do not drag your skin along the sheets.
- Use pillows to stop your knees and ankles touching each other, especially when you are lying on your side.
- There are various types of elbow and heel protectors – ask your doctor or nurse for advice.
- Using a simple bed cradle or duvet instead of heavy blankets can relieve pressure on your knees, ankles and heels, and make moving easier. Again, ask for advice.

- Avoid sheets made of synthetic materials like nylon because they are more likely to make your skin hot and sticky. Change your sheets often, especially if you sweat a lot.
- Take special care to avoid creases or crumbs in bed covers and sheets.
- If you sit up in bed, make sure you do not slide down because this can drag on your heels and bottom. Ask a nurse or physiotherapist for advice on the best position for sitting up.
- You might need a special bed or mattress. Your nurse or occupational therapist will tell you what is suitable and how you can get it.

---

**Carers** If you are looking after someone who cannot change position themselves, find out how to lift and move them correctly. This will help you and your patient.

**If you are in an armchair or wheelchair:**

- If possible, try to take the weight off your bottom every 15 minutes or so by leaning forward and pushing up on the arms of the chair. Or you could roll from cheek to cheek for a short while.

- You can get a special cushion to relieve pressure. Ask your doctor, nurse or occupational therapist if they think you need one. Everyone who has a wheelchair should contact their wheelchair centre for advice on cushions.

**Try to take the weight off your bottom every 15 minutes or so**

**For everyone who is at risk:**

- If you think you may be at risk, contact your GP and ask for advice.

- Try not to drag your legs and arms when you are moving or getting up because this can damage your skin. Lifting your legs and arms means that you will not rub them. And it's better exercise.

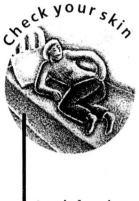

Check your skin

**Look for signs of damage**

- Check your skin for signs of damage at least once a day. Look for skin that doesn't return to its normal colour after you have taken the weight off it. For areas that are hard to see, use a mirror or ask your carer to look for you. Never lie on skin that is redder or darker than usual. Wait until it has returned to its normal colour.

> **Carers**  The person you are looking after may need help with this because the areas where pressure sores tend to develop are difficult to see.

- Keep your skin clean and dry.
- Avoid rubbing or massaging your skin too hard – especially over the bony parts of your body. Pat your skin dry with a soft towel.
- It's better not to use skin creams unless your nurse or doctor has prescribed them.
- Don't use talcum powder because it soaks up the natural oils in your skin and dries it out.

- If you suffer from incontinence, ask your doctor or nurse for help. They may be able to cure it. If not, they will be able to give you the most suitable things to make you comfortable. Make sure you keep as clean and dry as possible.

> **Carers** If you are looking after someone who is incontinent and cannot look after himself, always try to clean him as soon as he is wet or soiled.

- Eat a healthy diet and drink plenty. If your skin is healthy it is less likely to be damaged.

> **Carers** If you are looking after someone who cannot eat a normal diet, ask a nurse or dietitian for advice.

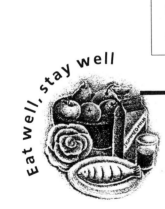

Eat well, stay well

**Make sure you eat a healthy diet**

❓ What should I do if I get a pressure sore?

**❶ Get professional advice quickly**

You must talk to your doctor or nurse. Pressure sores are unlikely to get better without treatment. Don't be afraid to be a 'nuisance' — always ask for help if you think you need it.

**❷ Eat a healthy diet**

It's very important to try and eat regularly and maintain a balanced diet that includes plenty of liquids.

**❸ Use the right equipment**

You can get a wide range of support equipment, including pressure-relieving mattresses, mattress covers and special beds. Your doctor, nurse or occupational therapist will tell you what you need.

**❹ Try not to worry**

Pressure sores will sometimes happen even if you are doing everything you can to avoid them. So don't blame yourself and don't worry. Pressure sores can be cured if you get proper treatment and look after yourself.

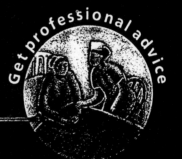

Get professional advice

**Don't be afraid to be a nuisance — always ask for help if you think you need it**

# Healing: a patient's perspective

A personal account of the problems of pressure sores and the importance of pressure relief in patients with paraplegia

Baroness Masham of Ilton, Ripon, North Yorkshire

**Pressure sores; Paraplegia**

In 1988, at the age of 22 years, and having just become engaged, I broke my back when my horse fell while I was competing in a steeplechase race. My back was broken at the fifth thoracic vetebra, which resulted in paraplegia, and I also sustained fractured ribs and multiple bruising.

I was transported from the racetrack in an ambulance and left on a trolley in hospital. I was in shock and in great pain and because of my paraplegia was at high risk of developing pressure problems. However, at the time I did not really realise what was going on.

I was fortunate in that, after 24 hours in an accident and emergency unit of a general hospital, I was transferred to the National Spinal Injuries Centre at Stoke Mandeville Hospital, near Aylesbury. I was under the care of the late Sir Ludwig Guttmann, a pioneer in the treatment of people with spinal injures resulting in paralysis.

At Stoke Mandeville, it was not long before I realised how important the three Bs were to any patient living with paraplegia or quadriplegia: bowels, bladders and bedsores.

Dr Guttmann would drum into the patients and staff that patients must be turned every two or three hours, and that this must be carried out continuously, day and night. How many times does a kind nurse think that it is better to let patients sleep at night and not turn them? And how easy it is for some nurses to forget that a person with paraplegia does not feel. We learnt to look for any red mark or lump or anything that had not been there before.

It was as a result of realising the numerous problems that arise for people with spinal injuries that I helped found the Spinal Injuries Association 18 years ago.

Our education at Stoke Mandeville Hospital was thorough, but I saw patients coming from places where the treatment had not been so good. They came from hospitals just down the road or across the world, if they could afford to come or their governments could afford to send them. I also saw patients who had been treated in private clinics who had been told that they were getting better. However, when they arrived at Stoke Mandeville, they looked as if they had come from a concentration camp; their bodies were racked by sepsis and their minds were depressed with the struggle for life. It was seeing these people that taught me that pressure sores can kill.

## Some nurses are not used to nursing patients on pressurised beds

In fact, in a survey on pressure sores carried out some years ago with the help of spinal units across the country, it was found that some of the worst sores were occurring in intensive care units of general hospitals.

When I left hospital and married and lived in Yorkshire, I often gave talks about the treatment of spinal injuries and how sport inspires many people with paraplegia to live active and happy lives. But I also came across many people who had had injuries and were having problems with pressure sores.

One young man whom I met had become tetraplegic through a gymnastic accident. Having been treated at a spinal unit, he was aware of what might happen when he was admitted to a general hospital with pneumonia. Such patients are particularly vulnerable to developing pressure sores. I received a note from him written by a student nurse: 'Sue, if you don't get me out of here, I will die.' I visited him in hospital, about three hours from where I lived. By now, his pneumonia cured, he had developed a serious pressure sore because he had been nursed in a ward with no procedure for preventing sores. There was only one thing to do — get him moved to a spinal unit, and this I did, with the help of his MP.

Sores will not heal unless they are clean and free from infection and slough, and the pressure is relieved. So it is vital that medical, nursing and therapeutic staff are taught how pressure sores can be prevented and how they should be treated if they do occur.

There are many technical aids available, such as turning beds, low-air-loss beds and many other mattresses and cushions plus beds made with Sorbo packs with spaces for the pressure areas. Some nurses who are not used to nursing patients on pressurised beds, and particularly patients who are also in head traction, are frightened of the specialised beds, but it is vital that they have adequate training in how to nurse these patients, who may have complicated sores.

Many years ago, I visited Mauritius, before it had developed its tourism and modern hotels. My husband and I stayed at an idyllic place miles from any town, the only medical presence being that of a witch doctor. I developed what may have been dysentery and for days I lived on the lavatory. I developed a pressure sore that would not heal and even after returning to the UK I felt unwell and could eat only soup and potatoes. I asked my GP for a blood test, but as he did not heed the results I had another blood test at a hospital where I had friends. I was told that I was anaemic.

I went back to Stoke Mandeville Hospital and was grateful for their expert help. The treatment involved having blood transfusions. Even now, I think that many GPs might not realise the danger of a low blood count in people with paraplegia.

Many years later, while evacuating my bowels, I felt something above my anus which had not been there before. I went to my GP who said: 'Don't worry, it is a thrombosed vein.' There was nothing much I could do. Some weeks later, when staying with a friend, I felt most odd, and, when I went home I discovered a small black hole. I contacted my doctor before returning to London and he wrote a letter for me to take to the A&E department of the Westminster Hospital.

I presented myself and the letter at the hospital. I knew that this sinus, unless dealt with, was going to beat me. I was examined and a swab was taken and I was told that I would be contacted if necessary. At the end of the week I went home to Yorkshire, by now running a high temperature. The hospital did contact me the following Monday and told me to come in to have the sinus dealt with.

The professor of surgery told me that the operation was only minor and that I would be out of hospital very soon. I told him that I thought he was underestimating the problem and, in fact, during the operation I had such spasms that I had to be held down. The staff did not expect this from a patient with a T5 lesion.

When I was back in the ward, the professor came to see me and told me I had been right. These devious sores, which infect one's system, can take over one's life. There comes a time when medical help is essential, otherwise they will kill.

After the operation I had to go through a difficult time of surviving in a general hospital without the usual equipment used for nursing a paraplegic patient. I had gone to Westminster Hospital because Stoke Mandeville Hospital had wards closed and an acute shortage of nurses. I felt that I did not want to take up a bed in the spinal unit when it was vital that patients with new lesions went there.

The healing of the wound was slow. The nurses were very helpful, and had to borrow pads and sheets from the maternity ward. There was only one lavatory that I could get into, and this was out of the ward and I could not shut the door.

The ward sister came back from 10 days' holiday before I left, and was amazed when

## These devious sores, which infect one's system can take over one's life

she saw that I was still there. She could not understand how long the healing process took. I went home after three weeks and the wound finished healing at home.

For years I had no further problems, but a small sore (from years before) began to give trouble. This was on my buttocks. I was vigilant, dressing it and keeping it clean. At that time I was going through a very busy period of work in Parliament relating to the onset of HIV and AIDS. I sought medical advice, and the staff at Stoke Mandeville Hospital said that at some time I would have to have an operation on the sore. The time came when I began to feel ill and I started running a temperature so I arranged to get the sore sorted out at Stoke Mandeville. No matter how busy one is, serious pressure sores cannot be left indefinitely. Their potential to interrupt life means they are something that every paralysed person dreads.

My sore turned out to be much worse than expected. But I could not be operated on until my blood count, which again was too low, had been improved. This had to be by blood transfusion, but this time the prospect was much worse. Having been involved with work on HIV (which was still in its early stages in 1984), the last thing I wanted at that time was a blood transfusion.

I had to have three operations, one of which involved removing some infected bone. After the first operation, my surgeon told me that if I had left it much longer I would not have survived.

The sore was infected with *Pseudomonas aeruginosa*, which meant I had to undergo a period of barrier nursing. I was nursed on a low-air-loss bed.

I was lucky that the antibiotics worked, and I survived with good nursing care. My blood took a long time to return to normal and the scar tissue has to be monitored all the time as the scar tends to get crusty. I rub in Vaseline or zinc and castor oil cream to keep the skin supple.

The subject of this article is wound healing, but I must emphasise that prevention of pressure sores must be a priority, as they cause inestimable misery to the individual and the financial cost to the health service is enormous.

I live in the knowledge that any sore may well break down if health problems arise. Growing older with paraplegia means that one must keep a watchful eye on one's health.

The great danger of sores is the toxins that are produced in the body. The other problem the individual faces at this time is depression — it can seem as though the healing period will never end.

I hope that this personal insight into the problems of infected wounds and the difficult task of healing them has shown how important it is to help prevent such wounds from arising, and, if they do develop, to see that they are treated and cured so that the person involved can continue a normal life.  ■

# THE PREVENTION OF PRESSURE SORES after hospital discharge

Moira Rough and Hilary Brooks discuss how

community nurses can prevent pressure sores

The patients most at risk of pressure sores are those with reduced mobility, poor nutrition, chronic disease or those who have experienced major orthopaedic surgery or major trauma and are elderly, although pressure sore problems are not solely associated with age.

Many acute hospitals now have tissue viability nurses and have, or are developing, pressure sore prevention policies. The policy at St George's Hospital, London, is particularly useful and highlights the need for district nurse

referral prior to discharge of patients from hospital.

If pressure sores are to be prevented in a patient it is necessary to assess that patient's risk of developing them and then to take appropriate measures to reduce this risk. In order to do this, an understanding of the risk factors and aetiology of pressure sores is necessary.

For example, a patient in a major accident and emergency unit may have been on a hard surface prior to admission, then transported on a hard ambulance bed to a casualty trolley prior to surgery on an equally hard theatre table.

During this time the patient may have been exposed to friction and shearing forces, enhancing the damage from direct pressure; within as little as an hour of hospital admission tissue damage will have occurred.

Correct lifting techniques and the use of pressure-relieving mattresses would have prevented this damage.

### From hospital to home

The discharge of patients from hospital should always be a planned procedure and care should be taken to ensure that the patient will have sufficient care at

home, that the district nurse, meals on wheels, home care, and equipment, such as commodes, will be available. Finally, the ward nurse should ensure that the patient's medication has been ordered. However, rarely, in my experience is any mention made of a continuing need for pressure relief.

Pressure sore prevention is an area of nursing in which the nurses should reign supreme. There is a wealth of literature readily accessible on pressure sore prevention and it is often the nurse, not the doctor, who is in the prime position for educating patients.

However, there may be some reluctance by nurses to report cases of pressure sores to doctors as the latter have usually

received little training on the aetiology of pressure sores and nurses may believe themselves to be at fault[1,2].

The preventive action required by acute and community hospitals and community nurses is essentially the same. The differences are:

● The types of patients and their assessment
● Having access to relief-providing equipment
● The availability of trained staff to ensure that planned care is carried out.

### Patient assessment

The assessment of an individual's risk of developing pressure sores may be scored by using a variety of methods, the best known of which are probably the

### Case history 1

An 83-year-old year old man who had end-stage renal liver failure and confusion was being cared for at home by his 80-year-old wife.

Initially there was little or no input from the district nursing service but the patient's wife made him stand regularly and took time to rub his bottom with cream 'to stop him getting sore'.

This may not be accepted nursing practice but relief of pressure combined with valiant attempts to ensure good hydration and nutrition prevented pressure sores from developing in this patient.

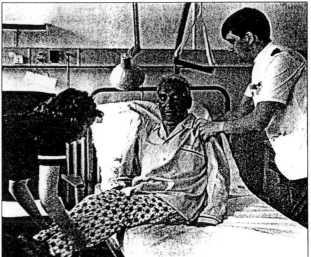

Turning a patient in hospital to prevent pressure sores

Waterlow[3] and Norton[4] scales. From this risk assessment score the nurse will incorporate the necessary pressure-relieving care into the nursing care plan. It is at this point that the acute hospital, the community hospital and the community nurse may differ.

Previously, in many acute hospitals, with the exception of medical and elderly care wards, scant attention was paid to pressure relief, and high-technology aids, such as the Clinitron Air Fluidised bed or the Pegasus Airwave bed were rented. In contrast, many community hospitals, well supported by local communities, may have had a range of low, medium and high technology aids and staff with considerable expertise in their use[5].

Changes in hospital care in the past few years have resulted in shorter hospital stays, and patients with high levels of nursing support needs being returned to the care of district nurses. Many community loans services have been ill-resourced to meet these needs, particularly in the field of pressure relief.

Both hospital and community nurses have often failed to recognise that patients in chairs also need pressure relief[6]. Wheelchair-users have long had cushions, and hospital patients with high-risk

scores may have the appropriate mattress on their bed, but chair-users continue to sit on unprotected armchairs.

The risk of an individual developing pressure sores is more likely to occur in hospital, as the reason for hospitalisation is likely to include the major risk factors, anyway.

Within the home when relatives are caring, there is one-to-one attention (see case history 1) and the risk of pressure sore development arises when relatives are unwilling to move the patient for fear of hurting him or her, but this may be overcome with advice and the use of a specialist mattress.

In residential homes, problems with pressure care seem more likely to relate to staff who are inexperienced and unaware of the need to seek nursing or medical help (see case history 2).

## Communication in continuing care

Good communication between nurses in the hospital and in the community is essential if pressure sores are to be prevented. But good communication requires work, trust and respect — it does not just happen. There must be an understanding of the acute hospital working pattern and its limitations, the role of the com-

munity hospital and the link role of the district nurse. In this way it can be ensured that patients will receive the right care.

Plans to discharge patients usually include making a pressure sore risk assessment. If further intervention is required on discharge, this information is communicated to the district nurse, receiving community hospital or home to allow resources to be allocated for that patient. In some instances the district nurse may require a detailed discussion of the case prior to the patient's discharge (see case history 3) to ensure that everything is available within the home.

The development of a pressure sore prevention policy to be used in acute hospitals and in the community, together with an equipment advisory team, would be ideal. Where possible, departments responsible for arranging equipment loans should have access to a protocol to help them allocate the correct equipment. They should advise the nurse of the most appropriate stock equipment and where to get further advice.

When problems occur with pressure sore prevention these may be identified by the ward manager and a bid made for the necessary equipment. Pressure

area care may then be monitored so that problems requiring action by hospital and community managers can be identified.

District nurses can give owners of residential homes advice on those patients who wish to be cared for in the home. In nursing homes, the inspection officer and community nurses may be able to develop good working relationships and share training.

## Conclusion
The prevention of pressure sores on a patient's discharge from hospital is an ongoing process. There are still many deficiencies in the setting up of care and the availability of resources, and there is a need for education and training in pressure sore prevention. The expense involved in treating patients with pressure sores has attracted a lot of interest both from the government and equipment purchasers.

References
1. Bliss, M. Death due to a pressure sore. Was the coroner's verdict 'lack of care' justified? *Journal of Tissue Viability* 1994; **4**: 1,10-13.
2. Crunden, E., Shaylor, S., Moron, G. et al. Step by step to a decision. *Professional Nurse* 1995; **10**: 6, 375–78.
3. Waterlow, J. A risk assessment card. *Nursing Times* 1985; **89**: 27, 49-51.
4. Norton, D., Smith, A., McLaren, R. *An Investigation of Geriatric Nursing Problems in Hospital.* Edinburgh: Churchill Livingstone, 1975.
5. Mack, S. Care and management of pressure sores. *Journal of Clinical Practice* 1986; **3**: 6, 219-21.
6. Gebhardt, K., Bliss, M. Preventing sores in orthopaedic patients in prolonged chair nursing. *Journal of Tissue Viability* 1994; **4**: 2, 51-54.

Further Reading
*Pressure Sore Prevention and Wound Management.* London: St George's Hospital, 1992.
Bridel, J. The aetiology of pressure sores. *Journal of Wound Care* 1993; **2**: 230–38.

*Moira Rough, BSc, RGN, RM, RHV, is hospital and locality manager at Walton Community Hospital, Surrey, and Hilary Brooks, RGN, DN, CPT, is district nurse team leader at Bournewood Community and Mental Health NHS Trust, Surrey*

### Case history 2

Mrs Smith, aged 83 years, was discharged to a residential home following her admission to an acute unit for treatment of a chest infection. She was not referred to the district nurse as it was felt that she was returning to a protected environment.

Although a care assistant was looking after Mrs Smith, she had no understanding of the problems that could develop when Mrs Smith became immobile and stopped eating and drinking over the following five weeks.

Mrs Smith then developed eight pressure sores ranging from skin reddening on the back and ribs to a black, necrotic heel.

The district nurse was finally asked to visit and made a series of calls over the next four days before a bed became available in the local community hospital. The district nurse had access to a pressure cradle (Karomed) mattress which stopped further deterioration of Mrs Smith's condition. Mrs Smith had a Waterlow score of 25.

The district nurse spent a total time of 12 hours with Mrs Smith. Time spent in telephone liaison and administration was five hours, and dressings on FP10 prescription cost £150.

However, these expenses do not, of course, reflect the unnecessary pain and distress experienced by Mrs Smith.

### Case history 3

A 12-year-old girl with a terminal condition scored 24 on the Waterlow scale and had non-blanching erythema over her buttocks. It was difficult for her parents to move her without distress, and a pressure-relieving mattress was required.

The problem was that her low body weight was below the recommended minimum weight for most equipment available in the community. The nurse manager advised that a mattress had been used successfully at below the recommended minimum weight on AIDS patients. This was installed and was successful in preventing deterioration in this little girl's pressure areas.

# PRESSURE SORE SUCCESS

Mark is paraplegic and has renal failure.
Diane Vernon describes care for his pressure
sore, including air fluidised therapy

MARK is a 20-year-old man who was born with 'spina bifida. The opening in his spine was closed surgically at birth and a ventriculo-atrial shunt inserted to relieve hydrocephalus. He is paraplegic and has a neurogenic bladder causing vesico-ureteric reflux.

In 1986, Mark developed acute renal failure caused by a urinary tract infection and septicaemia. He was treated with haemodialysis and discharged with an indwelling catheter but attended the out-patient department regularly so that his renal function could be monitored.

At the end of last year he was admitted to hospital with severe urinary reflux causing bilateral hydronephrosis and deteriorating renal function. Mark was prepared for renal replacement therapy and vascular access for haemodialysis was formed by means of a left brachial arterio-venous fistula.

Mark was readmitted at the beginning of February 1991 to our renal unit. He was anaemic with a haemoglobin level of 4.3 g/dL, (the normal range being 12–18 g/dL) and a large sacral pressure sore. This had been present for several months and it was being dressed under supervision of the primary health-care team.

The aim of Mark's care was to heal the sore, to be discharged to his family home where he lived with his mother and four brothers, to be able to carry out haemodialysis there and to be placed on the kidney transplantation list.

On admission, Mark had no idea how large his pressure sore was. He has no sensory perception of pain below the waist, but he needed to understand the importance of looking after and taking responsibility for his pressure areas to prevent the recurrence of such a sore. Factors which could influence the rate of healing were identified[1] (Fig 1).

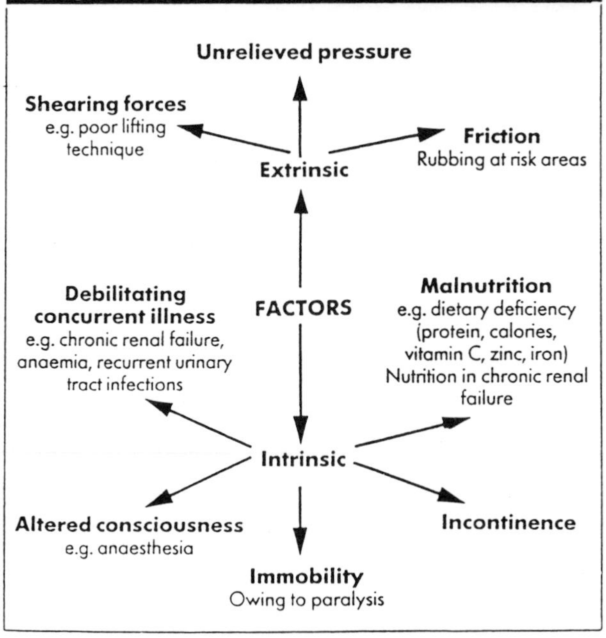

The sore was graded 4, as the epidermis and dermis were penetrated and a cavity was clearly visible[2]. The wound measured 18cm long by 9cm wide with a necrotic area along the top ridge, and a sinus in the middle. The deepest point measured 5cm, and some areas of yellow slough were present. The next day the wound was debrided. It appeared a pale pink colour and began to exude a pale yellow fluid.

At this stage of the wound management process, the use and effectiveness of particular dressing materials had to be decided, having taken into account Mark's particular physiological and pathological status.

Various research articles describe the characteristics of the ideal dressing, and the optimal environment for wound healing[3,4]. The ward team chose a calcium alginate dressing for Mark, which is indicated for use in heavily exuding wounds and available in a variety of forms[5].

The ribbon version was gently laid into the sinus. This was supplemented with a secondary non-adhesive dressing to absorb the large amounts of exudate, and we then applied a semi-permeable film.

A wound care chart was devised showing measurements, appearance, healing objectives, details of dressing and evaluation dates. The wound was photographed on February 20, 1991, a fortnight after initial debridement, to provide a baseline record (Fig 2). As healing began to take place we evaluated the amount of wound granulation and exudate. As these were satisfactory, with less exudate than before, the wound dressing material was changed to a hydrogel.

Initially, Mark was nursed on a silicone-padded mattress and then on a dry air flotation mattress. However, as the wound was producing large amounts of exudate, it became difficult to keep the dressing intact. This increased the risk of maceration and infection. The frequent need to change dressings disturbed the wound environment, thereby impairing healing.

At this point, a fortnight after admission, it was obvious some alternative form of therapy was required and Clinitron air fluidised therapy was chosen. It uses filtered air passed through soda-lime glass beads to create a fluid-like medium and providing patient support contact pressures well below capillary closing levels. Mark would be, in effect, suspended on a 'dry' fluid[6,7].

The factors that influenced the decision to use Clinitron therapy were as follows:
● Wound exudate would be easily absorbed through the filter sheet by the clinisphere medium, which is hostile to

**Fig 1. Factors significant in the development and delayed healing of Mark's sacral sore, using Morison's flow chart**

Unrelieved pressure

Shearing forces
e.g. poor lifting technique

Friction
Rubbing at risk areas

Extrinsic

FACTORS

Debilitating concurrent illness
e.g. chronic renal failure, anaemia, recurrent urinary tract infections

Malnutrition
e.g. dietary deficiency (protein, calories, vitamin C, zinc, iron)
Nutrition in chronic renal failure

Intrinsic

Altered consciousness
e.g. anaesthesia

Incontinence

Immobility
Owing to paralysis

**Fig 2. Mark's wound on February 20, 1991, two weeks after initial debridement**

**Fig 3. Mark's wound on May 16, 1991 after three months' healing**

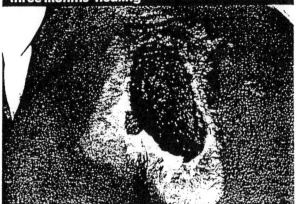

bacterial growth. This would reduce the risk of maceration and infection
● Less frequent changes of wound dressing would result, enabling minimal disturbance of the wound environment
● Mark could sit upright and be more comfortable than on previous mattresses
● He could move around the bed with the aid of a monkey pole, allowing him easy change of position
● Further damage to his skin by unrelieved pressure, shearing and friction forces would be prevented
● Continuous or intermittent air fluidisation permits easy change and maintenance of position when performing dressing changes.

We felt that Mark's sore would benefit from Clinitron therapy, which should allow it to heal faster. This in turn would, it was hoped, reduce the length of admission. The bed was hired from February 25, 1991 to May 3, 1991.

While we were making the decisions about the best choice of wound dressing and bed for Mark, the team drew up an individualised plan of care using the nursing process and Roper's model of activities of daily living[8]. The ward provides a team approach to care. The combination of the nursing process, a specific model and team nursing provides nurses with a coherent approach to care.

On admission, Mark was anaemic, a common condition in patients with chronic renal failure. It is caused by damage to the sites in the kidney that produce erythropoietin, the primary regulator of red cell production. Anaemia delays wound healing since it leads to a reduced oxygen supply to the wound[9]. This was corrected with several blood transfusions throughout Mark's admission and starting him on recombinant erythropoietin therapy, which helps to reverse anaemia in patients who have chronic renal failure and are receiving haemodialysis[10].

Mark had reached end-stage renal failure, so his kidneys were unable to excrete the waste products of protein metabolism. Without dialysis, these would build up in the cells, thereby impairing the wound healing process. Essential proteins and vitamin C are lost through wounds, and nutritional deficiency will delay healing. Advice was

received from the dietitian and Mark started a high-protein diet (60–80g/day). We also encouraged him to drink high-protein supplements.

Renal failure associated with the high protein intake he needed compromised Mark's renal function and he required regular haemodialysis therapy. A combination of dialysis, copious wound exudate, insensible fluid loss, along with the dry environment of the bed, raised the possibility of Mark becoming dehydrated. This was counteracted by encouraging him to drink and ensuring that as little fluid as possible was removed by dialysis.

Initially, Mark had an indwelling urethral catheter, but he suffered severe urinary tract infections. Antibiotic treatment was given, along with several changes of catheter, and eventually the urinary tract infections resolved. It was felt that the catheter was a source of ascending infection; therefore it was removed. We taught Mark how to perform intermittent self-catheterisation (ISC), but then he had dribbling incontinence, which caused contamination of his sore.

**MARK NEEDED TO UNDERSTAND THE IMPORTANCE OF LOOKING AFTER HIS PRESSURE AREAS TO PREVENT RECURRENCE**

On assessment, we determined that Mark was not performing ISC frequently enough, allowing a build-up of urine in his neurogenic bladder. We advised him to increase the frequency of ISC, but this was not totally successful. Although Clinitron therapy does absorb body fluids and the bactericidal action of the bed helps reduce the risk of infection, the situation was not ideal, as Mark still had a degree of dribbling incontinence.

Mark underwent bilateral nephrectomy surgery in April on the advice of the urologists and also in preparation for a possible future transplant. Clinitron therapy was beneficial in the immediate postoperative period. It helped to prevent further breakdown of Mark's pressure areas while he was recovering from a general anaesthetic and maintained comfort and reduced the pain which can be caused by moving postoperative patients.

Owing to his paraplegia, Mark had little control over his bowel action. During the first weeks of admission he was frequently incontinent of faeces which contaminated his sacral sore. A daily manual evacuation before performing the dressing helped to reduce this problem significantly. He also suffered occasional constipation, which was helped by encouraging him to eat a high-fibre diet.

Clinitron therapy helped to heal Mark's sacral sore in combination with the calcium alginate and hydrogel dressings. The amount of wound exudate lessened and the wound became a healthy pink, moist and granulated to surface level. Further damage to Mark's pressure areas and the newly formed fragile skin by shearing, friction and unrelieved pressure was prevented. This was extremely important considering Mark's reduced level of mobility, and it was vital during the postoperative period.

The only problem experienced with the bed was that it is heavy and not designed to be moved, therefore Mark could not stay on it during his haemodialysis sessions. He thus had to lie on his side on a silicone-padded mattress for four hours three times a week. However, this did not prevent his wound healing.

The cost of hiring the bed was high — approximately £4 000 for 10 weeks' therapy. However, if the therapy had not been used, the sore would probably have taken longer to heal, resulting in a more prolonged admission for Mark, which might have cost more in the long term.

Therapy was discontinued on May 3 and Mark was then nursed on a low air pressure flotation mattress. The sore measured 8.5cm long by 5.5cm wide and the wound was photographed again on May 16, 1991 (Fig 3).

Using a wound care assessment chart provided an easy visual description of the wound and details of the dressing. The wound was measured every two to three weeks but could have been assessed at weekly intervals. The outcome of evaluation was not always apparent and could have benefited from a better documentation system.

The calcium alginate and hydrogel products were appropriate and easy to use. When the wound was at its largest, it was difficult to keep the dressing intact. The wound was close to the anus, where it was difficult to apply the semi-permeable film. As Mark was also moving around the bed, the dressing occasionally became dislodged. Mark wore a pair of elastic pants to help this.

As a result of blood transfusions and erythropoietin therapy, Mark's haemoglobin level rose to 9–12 g/dL, improving the oxygen supply to the wound. (This is a satisfactory level for haemodialysis patients.)

The initial photograph of the sore was shown to Mark. He was amazed at its size and depth, and this realisation, along with having had to spend four months in hospital, has motivated him to try to prevent its recurrence by taking more responsibility for his pressure areas. Mark's sore continued to heal, and the focus of his care then moved to the preparation required for discharge.

On a home visit, it was discovered that indoors Mark was managing without his wheelchair, using his arms to shuffle himself around on his bottom. This was probably how the pressure sore had occurred. Mark spent a week at the local rehabilitation unit for disabled people for asssment of his mobility with regard to wheelchair seating and suitable protection for his bottom when out of his wheelchair.

He has since been discharged with suitable aids and returns to the unit for haemodialysis. He is now learning how to perform this treatment at home. Mark's case was very complex, making the holistic care we try to provide in our unit even more important than usual. **NT**

REFERENCES
[1]Morison, M.J. Early assessment of pressure sore risk. *Professional Nurse* 1989; 4: 9, 428–431.
[2]Lowthian, P. The classification and grading of pressure sores. *Care: Science and Practice* 1987; 5: 1, 5–8.
[3]Johnson, A. The economics of modern wound management. *British Journal of Pharmaceutical Practice* 1987; 7: 11, 294–296.
[4]Turner, T.D. Which dressing and why? In: Westaby, S. (ed.). *Woundcare*. London: Heinemann Medical, 1985.
[5]Dealey, C. Management of cavity wounds. *Nursing* 1989; 3: 39, 25–27.
[6]Turnock, H. Benefits of a bead bed. *Nursing Mirror* 1983; 157: 20, 32–34.
[7]Viner, C. Floating on a bed of beads. *Nursing Times* 1986; 82: 62–66.
[8]Roper, N., Logan, W., Tierney, A.J. *The Elements of Nursing* (2nd edn). Edinburgh: Churchill Livingstone, 1985.
[9]Morison, M.J. Preventing delayed wound healing. *Professional Nurse* 1987; 2: 9, 298–300.
[10]Winearls, C.G., Oliver, D.O., Pippard, N.J. et al. Effect of human erythropoietin derived from recombinant DNA on the anaemia of patients maintained by chronic haemodialysis. *Lancet* 1986; 2: 1175–1178.

This is an edited version of a care study which won the Clinitron Wound Healing Competition

*Diane Vernon, RGN, is a staff nurse, renal ward, Churchill Hospital, Oxford*

# The use of an airwave mattress for pressure relief

## A report on the care of a patient who developed a sacral pressure sore after being admitted to hospital with a fractured hip

Alice Jones, aged 68, was admitted to the female orthopaedic ward on February 2, 1990, following a fall in which she sustained a basal fractured neck of her left femur.

Ms Jones had a history of transverse myelitis — inflammation of the spinal cord — that had developed in 1975 and, at that time, she had been paralysed below the waist for nearly 18 months. This led to muscle wastage of the lower limbs. She made a gradual recovery at home with the help of her husband, a health visitor and a physiotherapist. For some time she used a wheelchair and, until recently, she could walk only with the assistance of her husband or by using a Zimmer frame.

Ms Jones lives with her husband in a three-bedroom house that has all the necessary facilities to assist life in a wheelchair. She had been walking with sticks for about one month at the time of the fall, which happened when she stepped on a loose stone.

As well as transverse myelitis, Ms Jones was suffering from long-standing urinary incontinence and she had a catheter in situ; she also had a history of occasional constipation. Ms Jones had experienced depression and had attempted suicide in 1986.

### Admission

On admission, Ms Jones appeared very nervous and agitated and seemed vague and forgetful. At this time her height and weight were not recorded because of her immobility, but otherwise her general condition was satisfactory. Her skin was clean, she was well hydrated and her pressure areas were intact. Her pressure sore risk-assessment score on the Waterlow scale, however, was 17, indicating a patient at high risk of

S.V.S. Rithalia, PhD, is scientific officer, Orthopaedic Mechanics Research Institute, University of Salford, Salford. E. Moore, RGN, is senior nurse, Department of Orthopaedics, Bolton Royal Infirmary, Bolton

**Pressure sore; Airwave mattress**

developing pressure sores[1]. Her clinical observations on arrival in the ward were satisfactory.

Following admission, Hamilton Russell traction with a 5lb weight was applied to Ms Jones's left leg. This was to continue as conservative treatment until February 5, when the fracture was fixed with a four-screw pin and plate. Pre-operatively her haemoglobin was 12.1g/dl. A catheter specimen of urine was cultured and *Escherichia coli* was grown. Postoperatively Ms Jones's haemoglobin was 10.2g/dl. The initial problem postoperatively was that Ms Jones became pyrexial with a temperature of 38.7°C during a blood transfusion. This was discontinued and her temperature returned to normal. Throughout the conservative treatment period and immediately postoperatively her pressure areas remained intact.

Ms Jones continued to make a good postoperative recovery and sat in a chair each day. The surgical incision on the left thigh had healed well. Unfortunately, an X-ray taken on March 4 revealed that the plate and screws had come out of the shaft of the femur. On the following day, Ms Jones was taken to the operating theatre for removal of the pin and plate. After returning to the ward, she was placed on Hamilton Russell traction once again to prevent external rotation deformity of her leg.

Until the time of her second operation Ms Jones had been nursed on a standard hospital mattress with a sheepskin on top, as a pressure-relieving aid was not available. Immediately after surgery,

redness of the skin of both her buttocks was observed, despite the fact that staff were using correct lifting techniques and Ms Jones was frequently repositioned in bed. By the next day a superficial skin break had occurred. One of the main problems now facing the nursing staff was the lack of pressure-relieving equipment at hand. Sheepskins were available, but there was a limited supply of foam overlays.

### The wound

A foam overlay became available on March 16. Over the next three weeks Ms Jones's sore developed from a very superficial skin break into a deep wound. Alginate dressings (Kaltostat) were applied and sealed with a vapour-permeable film dressing. Ms Jones was already taking flucloxacillin 250mg six hourly as part of her prescribed postoperative regime. However, the sore continued to deteriorate and, on March 20, the dressing was changed to a desloughing agent (Varidase) with a film dressing. This dressing was continued for the next two weeks when the film started to irritate the surrounding skin, possibly because of prolonged use. On the consultant's instruction, Eusol and liquid paraffin were applied to the now large area of slough, which measured 50mm x 50mm in area and about 30mm in depth. This dressing was continued until April 11 but with no apparent benefit.

The surgical incision on the thigh healed and the neck of the femur united with 4cm true shortening because of absorption of the bone. The pressure sore continued to get worse; it was now 75mm in length and 60mm in width. Polysaccharide paste dressings (Debrisan) were then prescribed. Over the following week the sore began to show

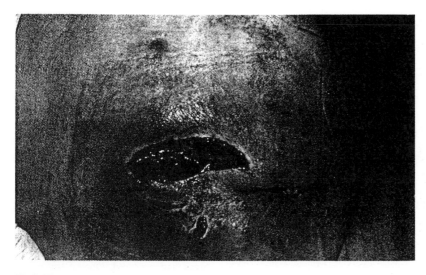

**Fig 1. The pressure sore before obtaining the pressure-relieving mattress**

signs of improvement, although progress was slow. On May 9, Ms Jones was taken off traction, which made it easier for the staff to turn her and achieve pressure relief. One week later, the dressings were changed to an alginate dressing. This produced a very offensive smell but the wound remained clean and its size unchanged. So far nothing seemed to have helped the healing of Ms Jones's sacral sore.

On May 17, the wound cavity was filled with a foam dressing (Silastic foam) and an alginate was applied to the surrounding area. A pathology report from a wound swab taken one week later showed growth of group D streptococcus, which was sensitive to chlorhexidine. On instructions from the consultant in charge, the foam was discontinued and, after cleaning, the wound was packed with gauze soaked in chlorhexidine (Hibitane). By this time Ms Jones had developed a very large and dirty-looking pressure sore.

### Treatment review
Having exhausted all the methods available at the hospital, outside help was sought which resulted in hiring a Pegasus Airwave pressure-relieving mattress in June at £67 per week[2].

From now on pressure sore management consisted of cleaning the wound daily by irrigating with normal saline and changing the disposable incontinence sheet, which was used because of the large amount of discharge initially produced. In order to keep records of healing progress, a wound-care chart was devised showing measurements, appearance, details of exudate and evaluation dates. The physical dimensions of the wound were taken weekly, across the longitudinal and lateral axes, representing the longest distance in both directions. Photographs (Figs 1 to 4) were also taken at monthly intervals to record the progress of healing over time.

Further damage to Ms Jones's fragile skin around the wound by unrelieved pressure, friction, and shearing was prevented. On July 6, Ms Jones was seen by the consultant in charge, who thought that she should start sitting out of bed in a chair. However, Ms Jones was afraid that her pressure sore would deteriorate and we decided to leave her in bed on the pressure-relieving mattress. Over the next three weeks the improvement to her wound allowed her to begin a programme of exercises and physiotherapy while lying on the bed. We obtained on trial a pressure-relieving chair and Ms Jones was able to spend a little time sitting out of bed. She was then able to begin to walk with the aid of crutches. The cavity slowly began decreasing in size and a month later the sacral sore was in the final stages of healing.

On September 14, nearly eight months after her admission. Ms Jones was discharged home. She had used the pressure-relieving mattress for a total of 11 weeks and, during this period, her sacral pressure sore completely healed. Thigh-length two-way stretch elastic stockings were ordered for her in case she developed swelling of the legs while walking at home. She was also given a device to raise the left shoe 4cm at the heel, tapering to 2cm at the toe.

### Discussion
The prevelance and onset of pressure sores in patients with orthopaedic surgical problems is probably higher than in any other specialty. This problem mainly affects older patients who are admitted either for elective hip surgery or with a fractured neck of the femur following a fall[3,4]. These patients often spend long periods lying on operating tables and in traction. They are often left undisturbed on hospital trolleys for hours[5]. They are also likely to suffer skin tissue trauma when left lying on the floor after a fall in their

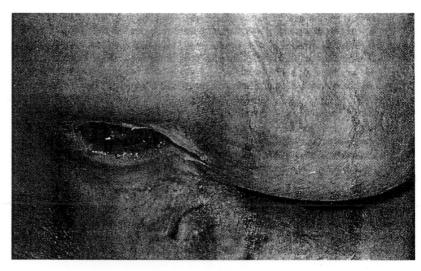

**Fig 2. After four weeks of treatment the wound had granulated well and reduced in size**

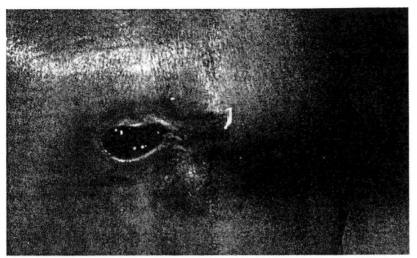

**Fig 3. Two months after starting the treatment, there was a marked decrease in the size of the wound**

own homes and during transport to the hospital in an ambulance. Furthermore, many elderly people are prone to a high incidence of pressure sores because of such factors as malnutrition, immobility and poor skin perfusion.

Pressures between the bony prominences and a conventional hospital bed mattress have been found to be unacceptably high[6]. Similarly, operating table pads and trolley mattresses create intense localised pressure[7]. Foam overlays and sheepskins are not adequate aids for the prevention of pressure sores in patients at high risk of their development[8]. In view of the predisposing factors, including a Waterlow score of 17, it was not surprising that Ms Jones developed a large sacral pressure sore. The wound had been treated initially with various agents including Kaltostat, Debrisan and Hibitane. Eusol and liquid paraffin had also been used, but as they occasionally came in contact with healthy granulating and fragile skin, unnecessary tissue trauma was caused (Fig 1). After the experience of treating Ms Jones a decision was made not to use paraffin and Eusol, paying heed to the well-documented research stating its harmful effects[9,10].

Before the pressure-relieving mattress was used nothing seemed to have helped in healing the sacral sore, probably because the underlying cause, the localised concentration of pressure at the sacrum, was not removed. However, quite dramatic improvement was noticed in healing progress within days of changing the patient over from the conventional mattress to the Pegasus Airwave System.

There was no need to turn the patient frequently and the mattress was easy to clean. Apart from irrigating the wound with normal saline, no other treatment methods were used on the wound during the 11 weeks it took to heal the sore completely. Undoubtedly the patient had also benefited from using the combination of a pressure-relieving mattress and chair.

The provision of suitable support surfaces for patients is a vital component in the prevention and treatment of pressure sores. Any patient requiring pressure relief in bed should also have protection when sitting in a chair. The Pegasus Airwave System in combination with a pressure-relieving chair had been of benefit in the treatment of Ms Jones's large and deep sacral pressure sore. However, the high cost of the mattress (£3350 or £67 per week rental) is likely to preclude its widespread use when other, cheaper support surfaces for pressure sores are commercially available[11,12]. ∎

REFERENCES
[1] Waterlow, J. Pressure sores: a risk assessment card. *Nurs Times* 1985; **81:** 48, 49–55.
[2] Livesley, B. Airwaves take the pressure. *Nurs Times* 1986; **82:** 32, 67–71.
[3] Versluysen, M. Pressure sores in elderly patients: the epidemiology related to hip operations. *J Bone Joint Surg* 1985; **67B:** 10–13.
[4] Hawthorn, P.J., Nyquist, R. The incidence of pressure sores amongst a group of elderly patients with fractured neck of the femur. *Care Sci Prac* 1988; **6:** 3–7.
[5] Versluysen, M. How elderly patients with femoral fracture develop pressure sores in hospital. *Br Med J* 1986; **292:** 1311–1313.
[6] Redfern, S.J., Jeneid, P.A., Gillingham, M.E. Local pressures with 10 types of patient support systems. *Lancet* 1973; **2:** 277–280.
[7] Gorton, B.S., Driscoll, P.A., Rithalia, S. Comparison of pressure distribution in hospital trolley mattresses and overlays. *J Tissue Viability* 1993; **3:** 33–34.
[8] Clark, M., Rowland, L.B. Preventing pressure sores: matching patient and mattress using interface pressure measurements. *Decubitus* 1989; **2:** 34–39.
[9] Thomas, S. Evidence fails to justify use of hypochlorite. *J Tissue Viability* 1993; **1:** 9–10.
[10] Moore, D. Hypochlorites: a review of the evidence. *J Wound Care* 1992; **1:** 4, 44–53.
[11] Bliss, M., Thomas, J.M. Clinical trials with budgetary implications: establishing randomised trials of pressure-relieving aids. *Prof Nurse* 1993; **8:** 292–296.
[12] Dunford, C. A clinical evaluation of the Nimbus dynamic flotation system. *J Tissue Viability* 1991; **1:** 75–78.

This article is based on an entry in the 1993 *Journal of Wound Care*/Pegasus Airwave Ltd Awards.

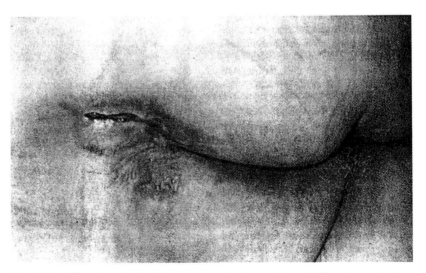

**Fig 4. After 11 weeks of using the pressure-relieving mattress, Ms Jones's sore had almost healed**

# A barrier to continuity of care
## Effects of the Drug Tariff on wound care in the community

*In light of the recent implementation of the Community Care Act, it is paradoxical that many products and dressings needed by community nurses are not available to them. This causes particular problems for patients discharged from hospital requiring continuity of wound care. What can be done to improve community nurses' access to the full range of products?*

**SANDY PHILLIPS**
SEN
*Community Nurse, Clwyd*

**JENNI FROST**
BNurs, RGN, RM, DipN, PGCEA, RNT
*Nurse Lecturer, University of Wales, Bangor; Member of UKCC*

In line with the changes brought about by White Paper 10 (DoH, 1992), 'quality' and 'standards of care' have become fashionable bywords among health professionals working at the cutting edge of the NHS. The Patient's Charter empowers patients to expect a quality service and choice through accurate information-giving – quintessentially the right 'to receive the right kind of service at the right place'.

Despite these developments, the government allows a paradox in the management of many community clients, particularly those requiring wound care, which denies them access to the most appropriate dressing products, and often breaks the continuity of care they received in hospital. This paradox is the Drug Tariff or FP10, the list of products available to GPs to prescribe and therefore, ultimately, to district nurses. The Tariff was devised by government to save money by restricting the products available on prescription through GPs – initially to encourage the use of more generics. Decisions about what to include on this formulary are not made by practising clinical advisors but by civil servants. Even though clinical trials have proven many products to be cost-efficient, as well as effective, the 'inclusion goal posts' seem to move (Dealy, 1993), and there is no recognised process through which manufacturers can get their products included. Meanwhile, pressures to reduce hospital waiting lists, accompanied by the increase of day surgery, have seen a quicker turnover and discharge of patients into the community, resulting in district nurses caring for an increasing number of complex wounds without the necessary resources (Dealey, 1993).

## Continuity of care – fact or fiction?

A great deal of literature emphasises the problems arising from inadequate discharge planning, particularly with regard to poor communication or lack of information received by community nurses (eg, O'Leary and Thacker, 1985; Sequeira, 1991) and its effect on clients and their relatives/carers. This situation may improve if hospital staff started thinking in terms of referring people back into the community, rather than in terms of discharging them (Saddington, 1985). Unfortunately, literature regarding the effect of the FP10 on the situation, or even acknowledging that a problem exists, is sparse.

Difficulties arise when people are discharged or referred to a community nurse for continuation of wound management, and the dressings commenced in the hospital are not available in the community. Do house officers prescribing the treatment, ward nurses or pharmacists realise there may be a problem following discharge? Do they care whether the 'good work' they have performed is carried on in the community once the patient leaves their ward?

The practical defects of this situation can be illustrated by the example of Mrs Smith, an elderly lady with a chronic leg ulcer who was recently discharged with only seven days supply of Improved Formulation Granuflex 20cm x 20cm. During her stay in hospital, progress had been good, but this particular size and type of Granuflex was at the time not available on the FP10, so Mrs Smith's GP was forced to prescribe an alternative compromising treatment by trying smaller available pieces of overlapping Standard Granuflex. Client compliance is essential for the management of wounds and the subsequent recovery rate. The amount of odorous exudate, strike-through and discomfort became unacceptable to Mrs Smith in her home, and her ulcer deteriorated again.

### Key points
Phillips, S. and Frost, J. (1993) A barrier to continuity of care: effects of the Drug Tariff on wound care in the community. *Professional Nurse*, 8, 8, 536-42.

1. Increasing numbers of patients are being treated in the community, with increasingly complex problems.

2. Community services do not have access to as extensive a list of wound care products as do most hospitals.

3. Hospital-based nurses are not always aware of the prescribing restrictions imposed on community services.

4. Healthcare professionals need to apply constant pressure until the Drug Tariff takes account of cost-effectiveness and a structure is set up for getting products included on the Tariff.

This case highlights the lack of continuity in patient care between hospital and community and, ultimately, surely leads to a second class service with respect to wound management. Not only do such incidents cause clients lack of confidence, disappointment and unnecessary distress, but they remain one of the most frustrating aspects of community nurses' work – particularly the lack of access to many of the highly effective modern wound management materials for the clients in their care (Bale, 1988).

## Understanding FP10

Several questions need addressing in considering the issue of products available in the community (Table 1).

**Hospital nurses' understanding of and access to FP10**   In a small-scale survey of ward-based nurses, Phillips (1992) found many were unaware of the limitations to wound care posed by the FP10, and had little or no knowledge of the existence of the GP formulary. In fact, many of these nurses did not know how community nurses acquired wound care products – some thought they had a direct supply from the hospital.

Nurses have a vital role in ensuring clients are adequately prepared for discharge/referral (Malby, 1992), including the continuity of wound care. Griffiths (1990) stated that hospital and community care were complementary: "There is an interaction between them and the need for planning must be improved, so that the appropriate range of services are made readily available at the time of discharge/referral from hospital – nurses must be made aware of the problem."

Nurses who took part in Phillips' survey were keen to learn and even apologetic that, as qualified nurses, they were unaware of the problem. They showed great interest in a typed list of the wound care treatments available on GP prescription, with which district nurses must comply (Table 2), so lists were produced for each ward in the hospital. Nurses could then refer to the list before discharge planning, and it hopefully increased ward staff's awareness of the problems encountered by community nurses. Six weeks after its introduction, the nurses' response to having the list was positive: although this is a short timespan, and not long enough to fully evaluate its effect, referral to the list was nevertheless frequent. Nurses were surprised by its limitation, not only of products themselves, but also size and type of the product. For example, Granuflex 10cm x 10cm and 15cm x 20cm were at the time readily available on FP10, but 20cm x 20cm was not, nor were 'Granuflex thin' or 'Granuflex sacral', even though they were all easily available on the hospital formulary. The nurses found the list easy to read; the alphabetical system made access to products fast and efficient – a must on a busy ward.

**Why are hospital and community formularies different?**   There is no easy or direct answer to this. Locally and regionally, it appears whichever pharmaceutical manufacturer makes the best 'deal' or purchasing contract with the therapeutic committee achieves access to a particular district general hospital's (DGH) drug formulary. If community services will not require that particular treatment in such quantities to make it 'value for money' or cost-effective, however, it will not be added to the Drug Tariff; indeed, as previously stated, products often have research to show their cost-effectiveness, but they are still not added to the Tariff. This method of addition to the hospital formulary may be good for the local DGH, but is not in community clients' interest; it also reinforces the two-tier system in wound care (Bale, 1988). Only if the decision makers, both locally and nationally, recognise that this system is unjust can GPs and district nurses be fully used as valuable links in the wound healing process (Savage, 1985).

**Pharmacist checks**   Hospital pharmacists are theoretically required to note in a book when any TTO they dispatch is not available on FP10; this then forms a contract with that particular client, enabling the individual or a nurse on their behalf to return to the hospital for further supplies. This system may sound plausible in theory, but unfortunately it does not always apply in practice. Given the tightly budgeted, financially independent trust status hospitals, who will negotiate alternative procedures when a discharged/referred client can be charged to the GP?

- Is the Drug Tariff or FP10 list available to hospital-based nurses?

- Do hospital nurses understand what an FP10 is, and take this into consideration in discharge planning?

- Why are hospital and community formularies different?

- On dispatching 'treatment to take out' (TTOs), do pharmacists check whether the treatment is available on FP10?

- How will budget-holding affect future accessibility of treatment in hospital and the community?

*Table 1. Questions to address regarding the Drug Tariff.*

## Effects of fund-holding

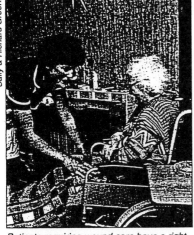

*Patients requiring wound care have a right to expect the same standards of treatment in the community as in hospital.*

**References**

Bale, S. (1988) A dilemma in the community. *Nursing Standard*, **2**, 17, 33-34.

Delamothe,T. (1992) The new NHS first years experience. *BMJ*, **304**, 7109-11.

Department of Health (1989) Working for Patients: indicative prescribing budgets for medical practitioners. Working Paper 4. HMSO, London.

Department of Health (1992) Patient's Charter and White Paper 10. HMSO, London.

Department of Health (1993) Personal communication; ref ADT/8/11, February 1993.

Dealey, C. (1993) Seamless wound care. *Nursing Times (Community Outlook)*, **89**, 31-32.

Ferger, H. (1992) How NHS reforms will effect general practitioners. *Pulse*, **52**, 16..

Griffiths, R. (1990) Community Care: An agenda for action. HMSO, London.

Guerrero, D. (1990) Working towards a partnership. *Nursing Times (Community Outlook)*, **86**, 14-18.

Malby, R. (1992) Discharge planning. *Surgical Nurse*, **5**, 1, 4-8.

Merck (1992) Medicine Research Centre Bulletin, September.

continued on page 542

In Wales, the Welsh Office is responsible for the allocation of money to fund-holding GPs; this is passed on to the practitioners via the Family Health Service Authority (FHSA). Nationally, there were, at the time of writing, already 3,000 GPs caring for 14 per cent of clients under the fundholding scheme, with 2,500 more due to enter in April 1993. Ferger (1992) describes the 'lynchpin' of the reforms as 'a split between buyers and sellers' – the buyers (purchasers) being the district health authorities and GP fundholders, and the sellers (providers) the NHS and private hospitals and NHS community units.

The allocation of funds to GPs is currently calculated on a percentage of the previous year's expenditure; unfortunately, many fund-holding GPs are running over budget. They appear not to have been adequately funded due to inaccurate expenditure readings of the previous financial year. Delamothe (1992) states that fund-holding is so new that it is not fully understood, and will take at least three years to evaluate its implementation. This overspending on the part of GPs raises the spectre of further problems involving financing 'expensive' wound treatment. If people are discharged/referred from hospital requiring certain treatments, will GPs continue this care via the FP10 or may they be inclined to prescribe alternative, perhaps apparently cheaper, options? Some of the new wound dressings have a high unit cost, but can remain *in situ* for longer periods and cut down healing time. Is it cost-effective to have a district nurse repeatedly returning for redressings, when using an initially more expensive dressing would have prevented this?

After contacting the local FHSA, assurances have been given to the authors that the indicative prescribing amount calculated from the previous year's costs does not preclude GPs from prescribing exceptionally expensive drugs, but the FHSA requires notice of such items. Treatment prescribing may be initiated by either GPs, consultants or both (thus sharing the cost of the care). The Welsh Office's opinion regarding the lack of access to wound treatment on FP10 and the effect of fund-holding practices and the DGH on continuity regarding wound treatment was non-committal. Two further questions arise from this:

1. If additions to the drug formulary are made in consultation with representatives of the medical and pharmaceutical professions, do these include a community pharmacist, GP or practising district nurse?

2. According to the Welsh Office, where it is clinically necessary for a client to use an item which is not available on GP prescription (FP10), it may be supplied 'free of charge' to the client through the hospital service:

- is there a policy stating this?
- are pharmacists willing to supply treatment not initiated by the hospital?

Although as laid down by the Department of Health (1989), it is the responsibility of regional health authorities (Welsh Office in the case of Wales) to encourage the development of joint formularies between hospital and community, many districts have committees composed largely of hospital doctors to develop a prescribed formulary. Surely membership of these comittees should be extended to include GPs?

Discussion with a local hospital pharmacist revealed there is a policy that states that consultant-initiated wound management *can* be carried on in the community, and supplied directly from the hospital if the product is not available on FP10. In practice, however, only seven days supply of treatment is given to the patient, who is not informed how or when to obtain a further supply. Asked why, if a patient is known to require, for example a four week supply of treatment, this is not despatched, this pharmacist replied: "Regardless of the policy on despatch of long-term wound care not available via the FP10, still only seven days supply is despatched, as 'this is the hospital policy'." This seems somewhat farcical, especially in the light of the Patient's Charter.

If GPs contact the hospital pharmacist requesting a particular treatment which is not available on FP10, but in their clinical judgement is required, the request may be refused because it was not initiated by the hospital. This is contrary to what the Welsh office has stipulated. Indeed, Griffiths (1990) stated that there will always be multiple responsibilities for providing care, thus creating a system where local responsibility for delivery of community care objectives are clear beyond a doubt. Unfortunately Griffith's recommendations are *not* clear beyond doubt. There has been confusion and misinterpretation of policies, as shown by both the hospital pharmacy's response and that of the Welsh Office. Since recent evidence shows that most GPs, district nurses and clients were in favour of day case surgery (Stott, 1992), it becomes increasingly important to ensure the same wound care products are available in the community as are in hospital.

## A full range of care

References (continued)
O'Leary, J. and Thacker, P (1985) A blueprint for liaison. *Nursing Times (Community Outlook), 81, 19*, 40-43.
Phillips, S. (1992) Continuity of Care Relating to Wound Management in the Community: a survey. Unpublished thesis, UCNW.
Saddington, N. (1985) A communication breakdown. *Nursing Times, 81*, 9, 27-28.
Savage, J. (1985) The Politics of Nursing. Heinemann Ltd, Oxford.
Stott, N.C. (1992) Day case surgery. *BMJ,* **304**, 825-26.
Sequeira, M. (1991) Hospital-home transfer. *J. District Nursing,* **10**, 3, 14-18.
Thomas, S. (1992) Cavity wounds. *Community Outlook,* **2**, 3, 10.
White, R. (1988) Political Issues in Nursing Past, Present and Future. John Wiley and Sons, London.

The Community Care Act, which has just taken effect, will ensure a full range of nursing and residential care in the community, providing district nurses and GPs with an ever-increasing client group. This is an ideal time for the government to correct the deficits within the Drug Tariff, but it does not seem inclined to do so. In a recent letter to a leading manufacturer of wound care products, the DoH (1993) stated that there was little prospect of any products being added to the Tariff in the financial year 1993-94 because of the ever-growing bill for prescriptions. Given the increasing numbers of patients treated in the community, and the increasing complexity of their problems, it is hard to see how community care providers can give effective care and keep the prescriptions bill down.

The only way to change this situation is by applying constant pressure to those with the power to make the changes. Nurses and other healthcare professionals, both individually and as members of unions and associations, should ensure their MPs are aware of the situation and its effects on patient care, and that the Department of Health is pressurised until the situation is resolved. In the meantime, hospital-based nurses should be made more aware of the contents of the Drug Tariff. Care in the community should be equal to that in hospitals; if it is not, then care in the community is a hollow sham. **Ⓝ**

# Care management in the community: a case study

**KEY WORDS**

Team work, ethics, community care

**ABSTRACT**

The rhetoric surrounding the reforms of the NHS and Community Care Act makes much of the benefits to clients. The reforms have been promoted as a means of improving efficiency and making services more responsive to the needs of clients and carers.

A case study is described here and the issues raised are considered. The incident occurred in 1994, the year following the implementation of the NHS and Community Care Act. It shows lack of coordination of services and teamwork, a poor response to identified needs and gaps in service provision.

*Margaret Elliott, MSc, RGN, DNCert, quality adviser, Kingston and District Community NHS Trust*

WHILE MANAGERS WITHIN the NHS and local authorities appear to be collaborating, there are financial and organisational reasons why collaboration and responsiveness are not always apparent at grass-roots level. This paper explores issues that arose from the incident described in Box 1, in which a lack of coordination in care led to a patient developing a pressure sore.

## The macro-perspective

Developments in the NHS and social services have occurred in response to changes in the economy and society. The most notable changes are: the growth in the number of older people in the population; changes in the family structure; increased unemployment; greater disparities in the distribution of wealth; increased female participation in the labour force; changes in medical technology; an increase in medical problems and the development of organisations based less on bureaucratic hierarchies and more on networks. Changes in public attitudes mean more is expected of services.[1]

Traditionally, care in the community has largely been provided by women in families.[2] Demographic changes and the search for more productive uses of resources were the catalyst for the Griffiths report[3] and the White Papers, *Caring for People* and *Working for Patients*.[4,5]

The Griffiths report recognised that services should be geared to the needs of the individual and the carer, with social service departments acting as lead agencies to develop care management.

The NHS and Community Care Act 1990 incorporated the internal market vision within the NHS and social services.

Since April 1993, social services have had the responsibility of purchasing social care reflecting the assessed needs of clients and using care management as an appropriate means of achieving effective care.

There are contradictions within the reforms. The internal market structure is based on a business model where the expected outcome is profit. However, within the NHS and social services there is no profit made and there is a continuous drain on resources. The internal market encourages competition which can actually hinder seamless care and collaboration.[6]

The established management structure that radiates from government down to local services appears to devolve responsibilities so that local services can become more responsive to local needs. In fact, the structure remains centralised and limits local decisions through policies and resource allocation.

## The micro-perspective

For clients, carers and professionals, there are both positive and negative aspects to these reforms. The Act stresses the importance of collaboration and consultation between all agencies and the client and carer through care management.

There is an emphasis on individualised care packages where each assessment should be an objective statement of the user's needs arrived at without regard to the availability of particular services or resources. Users and their carers should be at the centre of the process.[7] It should provide a comprehensive and coordinated service for the client, managed by a single person, the care manager.

However, it is apparent that in this instance this process was not followed. The assessor manager did not undertake an objective assessment without regard to the availability of staff, there was no collaboration between the health-care and social-care services, a comprehensive service was not provided and the service user's needs were not at the centre of the package.

## The professional perspective

The problems highlighted in the case study appear to focus on the management of change, and two organisational cultures working together. Neither of the services appeared to comprehend the care management principle fully.

The home-care service took the lead, but did not communicate with the district nurses. They took a service-led approach rather than a needs-led approach, and their assessor's main concern was the allocation of insufficient resources.

Hudson's research[8] into the practical difficulties of achieving needs-led assessment showed that care managers found it difficult to change attitudes from a service-led approach to those of a needs-led approach.

It is often felt that it is dishonest to identify needs, knowing that they cannot be met. However, needs-led services cannot be developed if the needs are not identified.

The NHS and social services have different cultures. Within the case study, the cultural differences led to a lack of collaboration and teamwork, and a lack of

**Box 1: A shortfall in shared care between home care and district nursing**

In one area clients with health and social needs receive both district nursing and home-care services. A client was discharged from hospital to live at home with her partner who had a neurological illness. The district nurses were visiting twice a week to give advice and support to both carer and client on diet, elimination and rehabilitation. The home-care service was providing personal care daily.

An incident occurred where the home-care staff placed the client on the commode, then left the house to finish their day's work. They returned five hours later to help the client into a chair. As a result of this delay the client developed a pressure sore. The district nurses filled the gap in the service, giving the care the home-care service was not providing. They also had to increase trained staff visits in order to give wound care.

The home-care staff reported that they had not had time in their schedule to return to the client earlier. The home-care assessor manager agreed they had not had enough staff to provide the necessary care. The home-care provider manager said it was not the assessor manager's job to comment on the number of available staff.

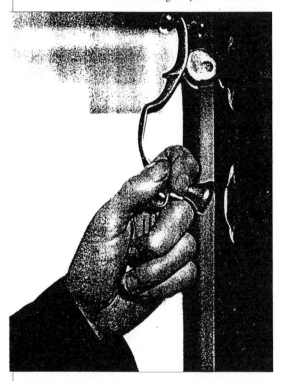

The director of home care stated that they had sufficient resources, but could not employ enough people to work in the early morning. They had therefore been employing agency staff, but the regular staff had not been working with them as a team. The district nurses and the home-care team had not been meeting regularly, coordinating care or sharing information.

The carer lodged a complaint about the home-care service with the director of social services and was subsequently provided with more appropriate care services

understanding of each other's roles. These factors meant that there were no joint assessments or meetings.

Because of the threat of role erosion, protection of professional boundaries took place. In the district nursing service this is represented by nurses passing assessment and care-management decisions to non-medical staff,[9] which happened in this instance. However, they did not initiate meetings to identify carers' training needs or share their knowledge about the roles they were handing over. Neither did the home-care service discuss the identification of district nursing as a lead agency in its own right.

This case study raises questions about where health care ends and social care begins and what shared care is. The home-care department and the primary-care department concerned had issued a joint protocol outlining how shared care would work but a gap in provision still arose.

Both services needed to change attitudes in order to become more flexible and 'user-responsive'. The Audit Commission has recommended that a designated person should manage the implementation of community care and that clear goals, appropriate training and involvement of staff should be in place.[10]

### The ethical perspective

The welfare state is based on certain principles: equity (equal care for equal need); comprehensiveness (providing a full range of services); and equality of access (care and treatment is not denied because of inability to pay). These values embrace the ethical concepts of distributive justice, utility, rights, altruism and economic rationality.[11] Principles of cost-containment and efficiency have been effective in social services for far longer than in the NHS.

One of the issues raised in this case study is concerned with rationing services and setting priorities. Both services have to undertake this process.

The home-care department's initial failure to provide a service has some basis in a utilitarian set of values. The district nursing service, providing social care at extra cost which it was not obliged to do, was following a rights-based ethic. One of the major stresses in the rationing process is the conflict between utilitarian and rights-based values.

The user-centred values of the community care reforms are to be welcomed, but at present appear to have empowered purchasers and not consumers. If the government wishes to empower users then public participation processes must be established. At a local level, staff need training in care management and the understanding of consumerism. **NT**

REFERENCES
[1]Ham, C., Appleby, J. *The Future Direction of the NHS.* Birmingham: National Association of Health Authorities and Trusts, 1993.
[2]Henwood, M. *Through a Glass Darkly. Community Care and Elderly People.* London: King's Fund Institute, 1992.
[3]Griffiths, R. *Community Care: Agenda for Action.* London: HMSO, 1988.
[4]Department of Health. *Caring for people: Community Care in the Next Decade and Beyond* London: HMSO, 1989.
[5]Secretaries of State for Health, Wales, Northern Ireland and Scotland. *Working for Patients.* London: HMSO, 1989.
[6]British Medical Association. *Special Report of the Council of the British Medical Association on the Government's White Paper, Working for Patients.* London: BMA, 1989.
[7]Health Committee. *Sixth Report. Community Care: The Way Forward.* London: HMSO, 1993.
[8]Hudson, H. Needs-led assessment: nice idea, shame about the reality? *Health and Social Care in the Community* 1993;1: 2, 115–123.
[9]Caldock, K. The community care White Paper: a nursing perspective. *British Journal of Nursing* 1993; 2 : 11, 592–596.
[10]Audit Commission. *The Community Revolution: Personal Social Services and Community Care.* London: HMSO, 1992.
[11]Institute of Health Services Management Policy Unit. *Future Health Care Options. Final Report.* London: IHSM, 1993.

# Implementing Nursing Research in a Critical Care Setting

*by Christine Breu and Kathleen Dracup*

During the last decade the nursing literature has contained numerous articles and editorials describing the gap between research, practice and education. For many people nursing research is of little value unless it results in improved patient care in settings other than those in which initial research was conducted.

At the present time efforts to encourage utilization of research are being made at institutional, state and regional levels. Although different methods are used to facilitate utilization, the goal is always to improve patient care through nursing research.

The content for this month's column is an outgrowth of a regional approach to facilitate research utilization. Breu and Dracup's exciting success story describes their use of nursing research to change nursing practice. It is one of the first articles on this topic to appear in a national nursing journal. The authors have every right to be proud of their accomplishments and of their contribution to the nursing literature.

**Carol Lindeman**

**Christine Breu, R.N., M.N.,** is a clinical nurse specialist in the coronary care unit at UCLA.

**Kathleen Dracup, R.N., M.N.,** is assistant clinical professor, School of Nursing, UCLA.

The Western Interstate Commission for Higher Education (WICHE) project was funded by HEW grant No. 00415, BHM, HRA, Division of Nursing. (Nursing Research Implementation Project)

In any profession the theory upon which practice is based must constantly be added to and strengthened. Most nursing administrators would agree that if clinical nursing research is not done and implemented our profession will find itself struggling with a no-growth phenomenon. But implementation of research findings is a difficult process. The nursing administrator who attempts it often finds himself or herself mired in countless excuses and rationalizations: the research does not apply to his or her setting; the institution is short-staffed; morale is low and it is therefore a poor time to institute new procedures; the medical staff is suspicious of changes; and so on.

The problem is centered around the fact that utilization of nursing research requires a change for all persons involved, and resistance to change is a normal human response. If nursing research is to be successfully implemented in clinical settings, resistance to change must be anticipated and planned for.

The column describes a personal experience with nursing research utilization, initiated for three reasons:

1. The staff of the UCLA coronary care unit where these authors work as a clinical nurse specialist and a clinical instructor had experienced long-term dissatisfaction in dealing with the spouses of critically ill patients.
2. The nursing staff expressed a strong interest in nursing research.
3. The authors were chosen to participate in a WICHE (Western Interstate Commission for Higher Education) project involving the utilization of nursing research. This project ran for six months and provided the authors with the necessary impetus and time constraints.

The WICHE staff also provided a framework for planning for, change that the authors utilized in planning for implementing, and evaluating the effects of change.

Based on the needs and interests expressed by the nursing staff of the coronary care unit, the study chosen for implementation was Hampe's 'The Needs of the Grieving Spouse in a Hospital Setting'[1]. This study was based on the theory of grief and loss developed by Lindemann[2], Engle[3], and Kubler-Ross[4]. According to these theorists, persons who suffer a significant loss, or those who anticipate such a loss, experience several common emotions. In her research Hampe studied the spouses of terminally ill patients who were experiencing anticipatory grief. The spouses identified eight needs which generally were not met by the staff. These needs were:

1. Need to be with the dying person.
2. Need to be helpful and of assistance to the dying person.
3. Need for assurance of the comfort of the dying person.
4. Need to be informed of the mate's condition.
5. Need to be informed of the impending death.
6. Need to ventilate emotions.
7. Need for comfort and support of family members.
8. Need for acceptance, support and comfort of health professional[5].

A control group of spouses of critically ill patients admitted to UCLA's coronary care unit was interviewed. These spouses expressed the same eight needs as did Hampe's subjects. Moreover, it was evident from the interviews that the majority of these needs were not being met successfully by either the nursing staff or the medical staff.

Because a change of approach was needed, an experimental phase was established using a specific care plan for the spouse formulated by the nursing staff.

In planning for the implementation of these changes, Kurt Lewin's force field analysis was used. According to Lewin, behavior in any institutional setting is not a static pattern [6,7]. Rather, it is a dynamic balance of forces working in opposite directions within the social-psychological space of the institution. The forces that tend to increase the possibility for change or movement are called *driving forces*. The forces that tend to depress change or movement are called *resisting forces*. As long as these forces are equal, the status quo will be maintained.

Change can take place only when an imbalance occurs between the sum of the restraining forces and the sum of the driving forces. Such imbalance unfreezes the pattern; the level changes until the opposing forces are again brought into equilibrium.

In attempting to change a situation and move behavior to a new level, three strategies are possible: 1) increase the driving forces by adding new ones or strengthening existing ones, 2) reduce or remove the restraining forces, 3) translate one or more restraining forces into driving forces. A change agent may use only the first of these three strategies, becoming a driving force by putting pressure on the system to change. In this case changes may occur, but it is often unstable and quickly reverts to the original condition. A combination of all three strategies is the most effectual means of effecting change with minimal tension placed on the system.

In planning for change, a change agent must take into account certain endemic factors that tend to work against either change itself or any effort to achieve it on a conscious, deliberate, and collaborative basis. Using Lewin's framework, Klein identified eight principles that we used in our implementation of a new nursing care plan for the spouses of critically ill patients[8].

### 1. There is almost a universal tendency to seek to maintain the status quo on the part of those whose needs are being met by it.

In applying this principle to a specific setting several assessment questions need to be asked. Is anything occurring in the unit that increases need to maintain the status quo? Have there been any major changes in the structure of either the unit or the institution? What changes are the staff trying to make in other areas? Exactly what kind of changes need to be introduced? What

kind of commitment and involvement is needed by the staff? What can be done to increase the desire to change from the status quo to a new level? What resisting forces are there? What driving forces are there?

When assessing our unit, we saw clearly that the tendency to maintain the status quo was heightened at the time we wished to introduce the project. The unit was very unstable because of a high turnover of nursing staff. In addition, the head nurse position was vacant, and the director of nurses and the director of the unit were both newly appointed. Furthermore, the sensitivity of the project and the energy investment it required from the staff meant that undoubtedly some nurses would not be willing to participate.

At this point a decision had to be made as to whether we were willing to invest energy to promote change at this time or if we should wait for a more opportune time. We decided to commence with the project, keeping in mind that it would be necessary to continually assess the influencing factors and to plan our approach around these factors with the utilization and application of change theory.

After identifying the causes of the unit's instability as resisting forces, our immediate goal was to decrease these forces whenever we could or to plan our interventions in such a way that they at least would not be increased. Realizing that good communication was of paramount importance in this situation, we met with all key people, including the supervisor of the unit, the new director of the unit, the chief of the department of cardiology, the assistant director of nursing, the unit leaders, and the ward secretaries, who play an important role in interacting with the spouses. In addition we had several meetings with the staff and then supplemented this verbal communication with several updates and explanatory letters. We attempted to keep all personnel informed regardless of their level of interest or participation in the project, hoping to prevent any interference with or resistance to the project by the noninvolved faction.

Included in the meetings and the updates was a reporting of the control data. This was presented in such a way that it helped the staff to identify the

nursing interventions in which they were proficient and those in which they could improve. We hoped that this would act as a stimulus to the staff to increase their interest and involvement. The control data also reinforced a driving force that we identified; namely, that the problem of dealing with the grieving spouses occurs frequently in the unit, and this in itself served as an impetus to change.

### 2. Resistance to change increases in proportion to the degree in which it is perceived as a threat.

In evaluating a situation with this guideline in mind one must consider: In what ways will this change, or process of implementing the change, be a threat to the staff? What does the staff stand to lose with the change? In what ways can one minimize or eliminate the felt threat? In what ways can one support the staff during the process of change?

Much of the threat that we identified centered around the uncomfortableness of the staff in dealing with this sensitive subject, which meant not only helping others with death and their associated grief, but also facing and dealing with their own feelings toward death. We held several sessions with the staff to discuss grief and loss theory, how it applied to the spouses, and to identify appropriate nursing interventions to meet the spouses' needs. This approach tended to increase their knowledge and confidence in dealing with the spouse, and therefore to decrease their felt threat. Throughout the study, we allowed the staff to verbalize both negative and positive aspects of their involvement with the families, supporting them and their efforts as much as possible. We used the control data in such a way as to commend the staff for areas in which they were effective, while maintaining a nonjudgmental attitude in discussing the areas in which they needed improvement. These approaches were used in an attempt to decrease the threat felt by the staff when dealing with this sensitive and difficult area.

The staff's general unfamiliarity with nursing research could in itself be perceived by them as threatening. Appreciating this resisting force, our strategy was to decrease this threat by reinforcing the goals, objectives, and methodology of the research and to provide explanations and informal education as needed.

### 3. Resistance to change increases in direct response to pressure to change.

To incorporate this prescription into the planning of change one needs to ask: What kind of pressure do the planners for change have on them to institute the proposed change? What roles do the principal planners play in the change setting? To what degree do the participants have a choice in the change?

As a clinical specialist in the unit, one of us had formally delegated authority, whereas the other as a clinical instructor had informal authority. Because of this authority, we identified our roles as possible resisting forces tending to increase the pressure on the staff to change. We attempted to decrease the felt pressure by emphasizing the voluntary nature of the project, and by accepting staff refusal to participate in a nonjudgmental manner. In addition, we encouraged assigning spouses only to those nurses who were willing to be involved in the research.

### 4. Resistance to change decreases when it is perceived as being reinforced by trusted others, such as high-prestige figures, those whose judgement is respected, people of like mind.

Questions to be answered when evaluating with this guideline are the following: Who has formal and/or informal authority in the setting? Whom does the staff trust? How can support from these individuals be elicited? In what ways can continuous communication with commitment from this group be assured?

We recognized that the unit was unstable because of a great changeover among key personnel. Consequently, we attempted to communicate with and gain the support of everyone who had authority and was trusted by the staff. No resisting force was felt from the authority group even if open support was not seen. We attributed this to our efforts to maintain open communication.

In this particular area our roles in the unit were advantageous. Both of us were well known and respected by the staff, and were responsible for the unit: both had worked together for the unit prior to the project, and were readily accessible to the staff. We feel that the staff's acceptance of us prior to the proposed changes greatly enhanced the successful implementation of this research.

### 5. Resistance to change decreases when those involved are able to foresee how they might establish a new equilibrium as good as or better than the old.

In regard to this principle, the assessment must include answers to such questions as: What factors point toward the need for the change? Who has identified the need? What problems have the staff identified and which are they willing to work on? Is the proposed plan of change related to one of these problem? In what ways can the staff foresee the new way as better? Is it possible to utilize the concept of provisional involvement to help the staff accept the change? What will the staff gain by the change?

In our unit the staff frequently has to work with spouses and families of dying patients. They expressed their uneasiness, and they themselves asked if there was something more they could do to meet the needs of these families. This gave us a distinct advantage because they were already looking for change. Again the control data were used to personalize the study and to help the staff identify how they could improve. We also set up the change as an experimental phase of the project, giving the staff an opportunity to observe how the changes would work before permanently changing unit protocol. Our in-service classes also served to provide the staff with a review of current research and literature to help them see the proposed changes as a tried and approved better way.

### 6. Commitment to change increases when those involved have the opportunity to participate in the decision to make and to implement the change.

Pertinent assessment questions pertaining to this guideline would include: Was the need for change identified by the staff? If not, in what ways can the change agent help them to see the need? In what ways can the staff become personally involved with the implementation of change? How much flexibility do the change agents have? What channels of communication are needed to receive staff input regarding the change?

In this situation, staff participation was high because it was from their request to implement change that the project got its start. From the beginning we also tried to give the staff credit and personal responsibility for the project, to increase their feelings of participation. All of the ideas for the interventions and the specifics of the planned change came directly from the staff. Because not all of them could attend these sessions to formulate the spouse's care plan, an update was circulated asking for further input before the care plan was finalized.

### 7. Resistance to change based on fear of the new circumstance is decreased when those involved have the opportunity to experience the new under conditions of minimal threat.

To utilize this principle, questions from the second guideline need to be expanded to include: What approaches can be utilized to implement the change and still maintain conditions of minimal threat? Does time allow for an experimental phase with the proposed change? In what ways can the change agents show their commitment to change and yet maintain a somewhat nonjudgmental attitude to minimize threat?

Again, offering the staff provisional involvement by means of an experimental phase decreased the felt threat. The staff know that they had the opportunity to try the change, assess the benefits and detriments of that change, and possibly revise it before adapting it into permanent protocol. Full involvement of the staff in developing the interventions also decreased the resistance to change because it decreased the threat of the interventions.

### 8. Temporary alterations in most situations can be brought about by the use of direct pressure, but these changes are accompanied by heightened tension and will yield a highly unstable situation.

This situation will not occur if time is taken to plan for change. Planning includes a thorough assessment of the potential pressures and threats that might be produced by the change, and of the appropriate actions that can be taken to avert these pressures and threats.

One continuous theme in the planning and implementing of our change was to keep it as nonthreatening as possible. In order to accomplish this goal we had to continually evaluate the amount of stress and the various factors producing it in our unit at any given time.

## CONCLUSION

We have attempted to share the kind of assessment that helped us as we planned for change. In our setting, we found that utilizing the results of clinical research added a new dimension to our clinical practice. Our interviews with spouses of critically ill patients following the staff's implementation of an experimental care plan were markedly different from those conducted prior to the care plan. Thanks

to the efforts of the nursing staff, the needs of grieving spouses are now met more consistently and completely.

However, such a change did not come about effortlessly. To effect change, a great deal of energy must be invested in thoroughly planning an approach based on a complete evaluation of the driving and resisting forces that exist in the setting.

Another important factor in this process is the nursing research study chosen for implementation. This research must be valid and appropriate for the particular setting. We did not meet the resistance among the nursing staff that might normally have been encountered, due largely, we feel, to our choice of a study that dealt with a problem already identified and given a high priority by the nursing staff.

Utilization of the results of nursing research can markedly improve clinical practice and add to the body of nursing theory. However, this process requires change, and change must be planned for and evaluated if it is to be effective.

The use of change theory can greatly facilitate the nursing administrator in his or her implementation of nursing research.

## REFERENCES

1. Hampe, S. The needs of the grieving spouse in a hospital setting. *Nurs. Res.*, Vol. 24, No. 2, 1975, pp 113-120.
2. Lindemann, E. Symptomatology and management of acute grief. *Am. J. Psych.*, Vol. 101, No. 2, 1944, pp. 141-148
3. Engel, G.L. Grief and grieving. *Am. J. Nurs.*, Vol. 64, No. 9, 1964, pp. 93-98.
4. Kubler-Ross, E. *On Death and Dying.* New York: Macmillan Co., 1969.
5. Hampe, S. 1975. pp. 113-120.
6. Lewin, K. "Group Decision and Social Change", in *Readings in Social Psychology.* Newcomb, T. and Hartley, E. (eds). New York: Holt, Rinehart and Winston, 1947.
7. Lewin, K. *Field Theory in Social Sciences* by Cartwright, D. (ed). New York,: Harper Brothers, 1951.
8. Klein, D.C. *Community Dynamics and Mental Health.* New York: John Wiley and Sons, Inc., 1968, pp. 123-126.

# The Nurse Formulary and Benefits in Practice
## *Sue Devon*

Even though the eight demonstration sites for nurse prescribing are all in England, discussion of the *Nurse Prescribers' Formulary* and the benefits of nurse prescribing is a relevant and useful activity for nurses and health visitors working in every country of the United Kingdom.

Several factors contribute to the different ways in which patients and clients in different parts of the UK obtain their drugs, medicines and appliances: For example, the numbers of dispensing G.P.'s vary markedly between rural and urban areas and items such as dressing packs, pads and special procedure packs are made available by some trusts to nurses via Central Sterile Supply Departments (CSSD's) whilst nurses working in other trusts can only obtain items on prescription. Most of these differences are historic and do not affect the principle of nurse prescribing or the content of the nurses formulary.

It is necessary to begin by clarifying what I mean by the term 'nurse prescribing'. The report of the Advisory Group on Nurse Prescribing (DoH, 1989) had as one of its recommendations: *'certain specified groups of nurses should be able to prescribe from a nurses' formulary'* and this activity the report called *initial prescribing*. Therefore, *initial prescribing* can be defined as taking place when an appropriately qualified nurse, currently a qualified district nurse or health visitor who has successfully completed an additional educational module on nurse prescribing, decides the item to be prescribed, writes and signs a prescription for a named patient or client and that prescription is dispensed by a pharmacist in a community pharmacy or by a dispenser in a dispensing practice.

### The Formulary

The concept of nurse prescribing came into focus as a result of being one of the recommendations contained in *Neighbourhood Nursing: A Focus for Care* (HMSO, 1986) now more commonly known as the *Cumberlege Report*. This report recognised what many community nurses had always known: that a great amount of time was spent by patients, their carers and their nurses in obtaining prescriptions and that nurses frequently had more knowledge of and expertise in the use of the items being prescribed than had the doctors who prescribed them. Creating a situation that the Advisory Group on Nurse Prescribing (1989) thought to be demeaning to both nurses and doctors. Members of the Advisory Group were nominated by the Standing Medical, Nursing and Midwifery and Pharmaceutical Advisory Committees and the chairman was Dr June Crown.

The very first draft formulary, which took many hours of discussion to produce was drawn up by the advisory group. Its basis was and continues to be items familiar to nurses and health visitors that are listed in the *British National Formulary* (BNF) and the Drug Tariff. The final draft version of this first formulary appeared as a list in *Appendix E* of the Report of the Advisory Group on Nurse Prescribing.

The next stage was the formation of the nurse prescribers formulary sub-committee as part of the implementation process of the recommendations of the advisory group. It is a sub-committee of the Joint Formulary Committee whose members are drawn from the British Medical Association (BMA) and the Royal Pharmaceutical Society (RPS), the two bodies who are jointly responsible for the publication of the *BNF*. The Health Visitors Association and the Royal College of Nursing work in association with the BMA and RPS to produce the Nurses' Formulary. The list of members of the Joint Formulary Committee is given in the *BNF* and the nurse prescribers' formulary sub-committee are listed in the current draft Nurses' Formulary.

The production of a nurses formulary has always involved close collaboration between doctors, nurses and pharmacists. Joint working between the professions has been a feature of all the work involved in the nurse prescribing initiative and its successful implementation will depend upon this collaboration being continued and extended to include managerial and financial colleagues.

*'The Medicinal Products: Prescription by Nurses etc' Bill* received its final reading during the last week of the last Parliament and the draft *Nurse Prescribers' Formulary* was ready for the proposed implementation of nurse prescribing in October 1993. The implementation was delayed but the formulary was kept in its draft form and has now been published with some minor modifications for use by nurses in the eight demonstration sites. One significant difference between the pilot edition of the formulary and the other formularies is the omission of the prescription only medicines because further secondary legislation is required before these can be added, but the principle that prescription only medicines should be prescribable by nurses has not been lost.

The draft formulary contains information about how to prescribe and about prescribing for special groups e.g. children as well as about any contraindications and side effects of the products listed. The formulary should always be used in conjunction with the latest edition of the *BNF* and reference is made in the Nurses' Formulary to the relevant sections of the *BNF* for details of all the products available, particularly in the wound management and stoma appliance sections. Briefly the section headings are:

> Laxatives
> Analgesics
> Local anaesthetics
> Drugs for the mouth
> Drugs for threadworm
> Drugs for scabies and headlice
> Skin preparations
> Disinfection and cleansing
> Wound management products
> Urinary catheters and appliances
> Stoma care products
> Appliances and reagents for diabetes
> Fertility and gynaecological products

The next edition of the *BNF* (28) will list the *Nurse Prescribers' Formulary* on the back pages using a similar format to that used to list the *Dental Practitioners Formulary*. The *NPF* is seen by some as very limited and by others as too extensive. Only time will tell which, if either, view is nearer to reality. Those working in the demonstration sites will be able to exercise their accountability by prescribing items for use appropriately and only prescribing those items with which they are familiar; just because a product is listed in the formulary does not mean that a nurse has to prescribe it. As items become available on the Drug Tariff and prescribable on the NHS they will be added to the relevant sections of the *BNF* and if in a section included in the *NPF* nurses will be able to prescribe these items. Therefore, it is incumbent upon every nurse and health visitor involved to keep up to date. Nurses who are eligible for prescribing should have no difficulty in fulfilling their educational requirements for PREP.

**The Benefits**
Reference has already been made to some of the benefits of nurse prescribing particularly its potential to reduce the time wasted by nurses, patients and carers waiting for prescriptions. Generally all the benefits are applicable to patients and their carers, doctors particularly G.P.'s, nurses, community pharmacists and the NHS.

The nurse who has close and continuing contact with a patient and who plans and carries through a programme of care is uniquely placed to make an accurate assessment of that patient's needs. The nurses' ability to prescribe items to meet that patients nursing needs would lead to significant improvements in patient care. The potential also exists to strengthen the nurse-patient relationship by allowing informed discussion to take place about treatments and the use of appliances followed by the immediate issue of a prescription.

Patients may be referred by others to nurses, especially when they require wound care or an appliance. Nurses will be able to work independently, assessing needs, taking clinical decisions and implementing care without referring to a doctor. This will save time for the patient as well as the nurse and doctor.

There should also be benefits for pharmacists because prescriptions issued by nurses for the items they understand and use may be clearer and more appropriate than those issued by doctors. There are potential savings to be made by more appropriate prescribing by nurses who have clinical responsibility for and relevant knowledge about the items being prescribed. In my opinion the already close working relationship between community pharmacists and community based nurses and health visitors will be strengthened and such relationships can only enhance patient and client care.

The possible benefits of nurse prescribing in saving doctors' time have already been mentioned as have the benefits in clarifying professional responsibilities. As with pharmacists, nurse prescribing should lead to improved communication between doctors and nurses as well as offering a greater potential for partnership in patient care.

Prescribing offers nurses the potential for enhanced patient and client care as well as the ability to take full responsibility for clinical decisions. Nurses will be encouraged to consolidate and extend their knowledge of those medicines, dressings and appliances which they use to complement and effect their nursing care.

There is a potential for financial savings to be made by allowing nurses to prescribe, but more importantly there is a potential to improve patient and client care. Even though the majority of community ,practice based nurses and health visitors are as yet unable to prescribe, there is some preparatory work that can be undertaken. Gaps in knowledge can be identified and rectified and new knowledge acquired. The draft formulary can be used by nurses as a basis for any contribution they may make to practice formularies. But probably most importantly nurses should make themselves familiar with the formulary and provide the editor and sub-committee with any comments they have to make about the information that it contains so that the formulary becomes responsive to those nurses who are going to use it now and in the future.

There have been many changes in nursing practice, medical practice and the structure of the NHS since 1987 and the publication of 'Neighbourhood Nursing', but the concept of nurse prescribing and the principle of initial prescribing from a single nurse formulary continue to be relevant. ✦

**References**
DoH (1989) *Report of the Advisory Group on Nurse Prescribing*
HMSO (1986) *Neighbourhood Nursing: A Focus for Care* (Report of the Community Nursing Review)

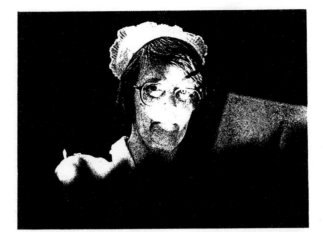

# PRACTICE THEMES

*An audit of pressure sore management practices in north-east
Grampian had the aim of improving care and providing a
baseline for future monitoring. Gail Field (above) explains*

TO promote good practice and
improve the management and
prevention of pressure sores in
community hospitals across north-east Grampian, it was
decided to undertake an audit to provide baseline information
that would assist in drawing up a policy on treatment.

The purpose of the audit was to obtain an accurate picture
of the nature and extent of the
problem across a group of
community hospitals. There
was no intention of having a
witch-hunt, nor of putting the
blame on nurses. It was
important to establish a team
approach, so initially time and
effort was spent on explaining
the background to the audit.

To ensure uniform grading
of pressure sores across hospitals, a definition sheet was
prepared specifically for the
study (Fig 1).[1]

The hospitals involved
cover a wide area of Grampian; the smallest has 11 beds
and the largest 73 beds (Fig
2). The specialties surveyed
included long-term care of
the elderly (both general/
mental health), acute general
practitioner and surgical,
where the hospital had a
visiting consultant who operated weekly. Nurse managers
were approached and trained
staff were asked to take part.

## PRESSURE SORE AUDIT

### Fig 1. Definition and classification of pressure sores

*Grade of sores[1]*

| | |
|---|---|
| Grade 1 | Discolouration of skin, with persistent erythema after pressure is released. (Balancing with light finger pressure indicates that the microcirculation is still intact). A blister may be forming |
| Grade 2 | Oedema, blistering, epidermal skin loss, with exposure of the dermis. Pain is present. Abrasion can cause this pressure |
| Grade 3 | Loss of tissue through the dermis, the edge is distinct and is surrounded by erythema and induration |
| Grade 4 | A lesion that extends into the subcutaneous tissue and may penetrate deeper into the deep facia and muscles. It presents initially as an area of bluish-black discolouration which turns into black eschar (hard black crust). After a few days/weeks, this separates to reveal an underlying cavity, formed by pressure destruction of deep tissue |

*Condition of wound tissue*

| | |
|---|---|
| Pink | Clean pink tissue which may be accompanied by healthy granulation |
| Sloughy | Tissue debris in process of being cast off |
| Necrotic | Dead tissue, brown, grey or black |
| Infected | Presence of pus, odour, inflammation, positive swab result |
| Exudate | None; slight; moderate; profuse |

A hospital not involved in the survey
was used to test the questionnaire
designed for the audit. The questionnaire was divided into the following sections: ward profile,
Norton score, patient profile and hospital pressure-relieving
equipment. The ward profile was filled in by each ward and
produced information including numbers of patients in each
ward and numbers of sores.

The Norton score section
was filled in for each patient
and recorded information
about their age, any pressure-relieving aids being used and
their score.[2] There were
three reasons for choosing
the Norton score:
● It is generally known and
was already used by some
wards
● It is quick to use
● The scale designed for use
with older patients was ideal
as the surveyed hospitals have
many elderly clients.

Section three sought
information about the types of
sore or sores each patient had
and their exact location; an
outline of a human figure was
used to record this. Section
four focused on the numbers
and types of equipment available in each hospital and
sought information on
mattresses.[3]

The audit was aimed at

measuring prevalence and had to be completed over a specific time (24 hours) in all the hospitals. I visited each hospital in the 10 days before the audit to deliver the questionnaire and to explain the purpose of the survey. Staff were asked to start recording information at 8am on a designated date and finish by 8am the following day.

The results were analysed on computer. As predicted, we found we had a large population of older patients — 8% aged 64 years or below, 14% were 65–74 years old and 77% 75 or over.

All patients with a score of 14 or below were considered at risk of developing pressure sores. Of 453 patients, 254 (56%) were at risk on the day, 184 (41%) scored 15 or higher and so were not seen to be at risk; 15 (3%) patients were not scored. The patients were also assessed at high risk if they had a score of 10 or below; at medium risk if they scored 11 or 12, and at lower risk if they scored 13 or 14.

The Norton score was the tool used in 11 wards and Waterlow in two; however, 12 wards did not use any tool.

The overall number of patients with sores was 102; they had a total of 167 sores, with 42 patients having more than one. There were 21 patients who had Norton scores of 15 or higher and were therefore considered not to be at risk, but who developed sores. Out of 167 sores, 27 were present on admission and 107 developed after admission. This information was not recorded on 32 (19%)

| Fig 2. Hospital population included in the audit | |
| --- | --- |
| Hospitals | 13 |
| Wards | 25 |
| Number of beds | 515 |
| Number of patients | 453 |
| Male patients | 154 |
| Female patients | 299 |
| Bed occupancy | 88% |

Sores were graded (Fig 3). They were distributed widely, with the main concentration on the buttocks, sacrum and heels (Fig 4). Buttock sores usually develop when the patient remains in the sitting position for long periods because body weight is transferred through the ischial tuberosities to the buttocks.[4] The fact that 55 buttock sores found were in this study suggests that our patients were sitting out of bed for long periods. This points to the need to consider the use pressure-relieving cushions. Older patients who are immobile and sit out of bed for long periods are more at risk than those who remain immobile in bed.[5]

Sacral sores often develop when the patient lies in a semi-recumbent position; shearing and friction occur because the patient easily slips down the bed.[4]

The audit showed that nurses chose most of the dressings. There was a large selection of lotions, topical applications and dressings in use (four lotions, 21 topical applications and 13 dressings), 33 sores graded 2-4 were left exposed and 35 sores, described as sloughy or necrotic, did not have suitable desloughing agents applied. Treatment of pressure sores was 'patchy'; Eusol was not used, but the variety of products that were suggested a lack of knowledge.

In all, 75% of decisions were made by nurses, less than 10% by doctors. In only three cases where responses were available was the decision made jointly (Fig 5). This

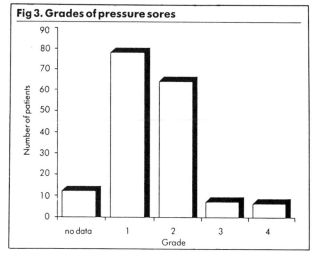

**Nurses chose most of the dressings for pressure sores**

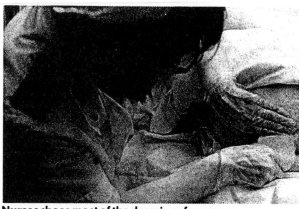

Fig 3. Grades of pressure sores

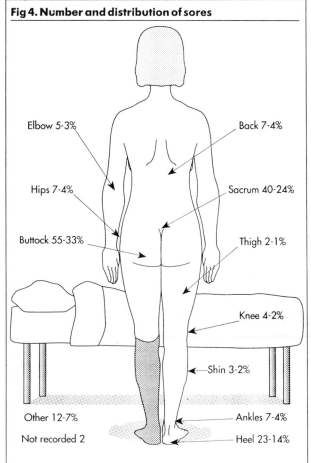

Fig 4. Number and distribution of sores

Elbow 5-3%
Back 7-4%
Hips 7-4%
Sacrum 40-24%
Buttock 55-33%
Thigh 2-1%
Knee 4-2%
Shin 3-2%
Other 12-7%
Ankles 7-4%
Not recorded 2
Heel 23-14%

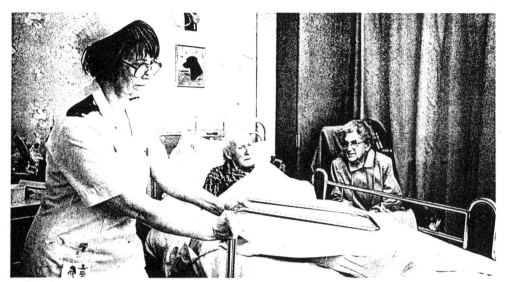

**Bed cradles take the weight of the bedclothes off a patient's body, easing pressure on heels**

heightens the need for good knowledge on this subject for all staff. More education will be needed.

A wide range of preventive measures were listed. The nursing care prescribed was categorised into six groups. These included turning and repositioning; ensuring an adequate diet and fluid intake; encouraging the patient to move about, either in bed or by walking; minimising the effects of continence problems; regular personal hygiene; and the use of aids such as hoists.

The audit revealed that a large number of mattresses and overlays were available across the hospitals, although not all were in use; six items needed repair, and one hospital had storage problems. Overall, 241 pressure-relieving matresses were available. Taking into account that 254 patients were at risk of developing sores on the day left the hospitals with a shortfall of 14. But there were also 21 patients with a Norton score of 15 or more with sores who also needed a mattress or overlay. This brought the total of patients in need to 275, with a shortfall of 34.

However, because 34 ripple mattresses and none of the net beds were in use, this complicated matters further, so the final number of mattresses that were available but not in use was 46, leaving 80 patients without a protective mattress. This had obvious implications for vulnerable patients.

It is therefore vital for each ward to use a scoring tool in order to determine which patients are at greatest risk and in need of pressure-relieving aids. However, the audit revealed that some wards did not use any tool. This is not to say that nurses' clinical judgement is to be disregarded,[6] but the use of a scoring tool on a regular basis provides objective evidence and assists in making difficult decisions on the use of equipment.

Patients at high risk were definitely not well off. They numbered 103 and only had 17 items of equipment between them. It became clear that 86 patients who were at high risk were being nursed without the aid of suitable pressure-relieving mattresses or overlays. At that time there was not enough of the right type of equipment in the hospitals. Since then the amount of suitable equipment has greatly increased.

In response to the audit, a multidisciplinary team has been set up as a pilot scheme in the Banff and Buchan District, which is part of the community division of Grampian Health Care. Its members cover a broad cross-section of disciplines and include link nurses from each hospital (Fig 6). Community link nurses from each of the four localities have now joined the team. The link nurses will seek to fulfil a similar role to that of a lead nurse in the ward of a larger acute hospital.[7]

The multidisciplinary team started work last January. A policy for prevention and treatment of pressure sores has now been drafted and should be in use next month. This provides for monthly re-auditing of the number of patients at risk of developing sores, incidence, grade and treatment.

As with all point prevalence studies, this audit gave a snapshot view of the situation at one specific time and for this reason its conclusions have limitations.

However, the results gave us a revealing insight and provided a basis on which to work. Regular re-auditing will give us the chance to draw comparisons and evaluate standards of care. **NT**

**Fig 5. Choice of dressings**

| Who chose | Number (%) |
|---|---|
| Nurses | 125 (75) |
| Doctors | 15 (9) |
| Both | 3 (2) |
| Not recorded | 24 (14) |

**Fig 6. Multidisciplinary team members**

- District general manager
- Quality development officer
- Senior physiotherapist
- Senior occupational therapist
- Divisional pharmacist
- Dietitian
- Project adviser
- Link nurses from each hospital and the four community localities

REFERENCES
[1]Hibbs, P.J. *Pressure Area Care for the City of Hackney Health Authority*. London: City and Hackney Health Authority, 1988.
[2]Norton, D. *An Investigation of Geriatric Nursing Problems in Hospital*. Edinburgh: Churchill Livingstone, 1975.
[3]King's Fund Centre. *The Prevention Management of Pressure Sores Within Health Districts*. London: King's Fund Centre, 1989.
[4]Collier, M. A sore point. *Community Outlook* 1990; October, 29–32.
[5]Clark, M.O. et al. Pressure sores. *Nursing Times* 1978; 363.
[6]Barrat, E. Putting risk calculators in their place. Pressure Sores Supplement. *Nursing Times* 1987; 83: 7, 65–70.
[7]Richardson, B. Lead role concept in wound care management. *Journal of Tissue Viability* 1992; 2: 2, 99–100.

*Gail Field, RGN, RM, is relief sister at Fraserburgh Hospital, Fraserburgh, Aberdeenshire*

# Assessments

# Level 2 assessment

This assessment is in the form of a 3000–3500 word essay (excluding references, diagrams and appendices).

The essay is in two parts.

## PART A

With reference to available literature, discuss in depth the scope and nature of pressure sore prevention and management, highlight key causes, risk factors and methods of prevention. This discussion should include government targets and any national or local guidelines and technological advances.

This part of your essay should be no more than 1500 words in total.

## PART B

1. Begin part B by identifying a patient in your care who is either at risk from pressure sores or who has an established pressure sore. Briefly describe the patient's potential or actual pressure sore problem and the causes of or predisposing factors to this particular patient's pressure sore. Remember to use a pseudonym to maintain confidentiality of the real patient.

2. Continue part B of the essay by undertaking a critical analysis of the assessment, treatment and/or support given to your selected patient. Your critical analysis will be carried out as follows.

   a. From the list below select **two** components of pressure sore prevention or management related to your selected patient:

      - patient's underlying disease/illness and its treatment
      - social/age/gender issues
      - nutritional problems
      - risk assessment
      - assessment of established pressure sore
      - nurse prescribing for pressure sore management
      - patient education for pressure sore prevention
      - ethical/legal issues in pressure sore prevention and management.

   b. Examine the interrelationships or connections between the two components you selected from the list above (e.g. how does component A relate to component B?).

   c. How do the components which you selected come together to influence the prevention and/or management of this patient's pressure sore?

3. Finish your essay by reflecting on the analysis of the care actually given to your selected patient, identifying what you have learned from undertaking this critical analysis.

This part of your essay should be no more than 2000 words.

## LEVEL 2 ASSESSMENT—MARKING GRID

| | Max. | Your marks | Min. | |
|---|---|---|---|---|
| Evidence of comprehensive discussion of the scope and nature of pressure sore prevention and management. Key issues identified. Discussion includes references to relevant literature. | 25 | | 0 | Superficial discussion of the scope and nature of pressure sore prevention and management. Key issues not identified and/or discussion does not refer to relevant literature. |
| Clear identification and brief description of an appropriate patient who is either at risk for pressure sore or who has an established pressure sore. Causes and predisposing factors identified. | 10 | | 0 | Clear identification of a relevant patient is not evident. Description of patient is absent and/or causes or predisposing factors have not been identified. |
| Two key components of pressure sore prevention or management selected and are appropriate to the chosen patient. | 15 | | 0 | Fewer than two components of pressure sore prevention or management are identified; or, two components are identified but are clearly inappropriate to the patient selected. |
| A comprehensive critical analysis is evident and indicates how the two selected components of pressure sore prevention or management are interrelated or connected and how the two components influence prevention and management of pressure sores in this patient. | 30 | | 0 | Superficial critical analysis of how the two selected components are interrelated or connected to each other; superficial understanding demonstrated of how these two components come together to influence pressure sore prevention or management. |
| Evidence of reflection on the care given and identification of learning which has taken place as a result of this critical analysis. | 10 | | 0 | No evidence of reflection and/or identification of learning which has taken place. |
| Essay is logically developed, within word limit and correctly referenced using a recognised referencing system. | 10 | | 0 | Essay is illogical, not within word limit, incorrectly referenced and/or does not use a recognised referencing system. |

# Level 3 assessment

Nurses who wish to complete this learning package and be assessed at level 3 can submit the following assessment. This assessment should be 3500–4000 words (excluding references, diagrams and appendices).

The assessment is in two parts.

## PART A

In this part of your essay you will identify one aspect of pressure sore prevention, support or management (examples: age and risk assessment; nutrition and pressure sore development; critical evaluation of different risk assessment methods; resource allocation and pressure sore management—these are only examples and you are free to select any other aspect of pressure sore prevention, management or support).

Give a rationale for selecting this particular aspect with reference to your experiences, government targets, the literature or local/national pressure sore prevention and management guidelines. Then undertake a literature review related to your selected aspect of pressure sore prevention, support or management, presenting in this part of your essay a critical review of the literature related to the aspect you selected to examine. In your critical review you should focus on similarities, differences, contradictions and agreements that appear in the literature. Justify your own opinions, suggestions and observations by providing evidence from your literature search.

This part of your essay should be no more than 1800 words.

## PART B

Part B of your assessment involves you planning a change to *your own* practice with regard to pressure sore prevention, management or support. Your plan should include the following.

1. Begin your plan by identifying clearly the change you wish to make to your practice, the goal or aim or purpose for making this change and the rationale for wanting to make this change. Your rationale should reflect research evidence, changing technologies, local/national guidelines or government targets with regard to pressure sore prevention, management or support.

2. Identify the timescale you think is appropriate to the change you want to make and justify the timescale. Indicate what you expect to be different in that timescale as a result of making this change (i.e. ask yourself, 'What will I notice or see in X months that will enable to me know that the change is or is not effective?').

3. *With reference to change theory*, present an action plan which includes the things you need to do to make this change successful (in chronological order), who else you might need to involve and by when each activity in your action plan is expected to be completed.

4. Again, with reference to change theory, identify any potential problems, resistance or barriers to successful change which you might encounter and the change methods which you might use to prevent or overcome some of these difficulties.

5. Conclude your essay by briefly describing how you propose to evaluate the effectiveness of your change attempt.

Part B of your essay should be no more than 2200 words.

## LEVEL 3 ASSESSMENT—MARKING GRID

| | Max. | Your marks | Min. | |
|---|---|---|---|---|
| Selected aspect of pressure sore prevention, management or support is clearly identified including rationale for selecting this aspect. | 10 | | 0 | Selected aspect of pressure sore prevention, management or support not clearly identified and/or no rationale for selection is included. |
| Comprehensive **critical** literature review is presented. | 20 | | 0 | Literature review is superficial and/or not presented critically. |
| Clear presentation of the change being proposed, including the goal or purpose and rationale for making this change. Rationale clearly reflects research evidence, changing technologies, local/national guidelines and/or government targets. | 15 | | 0 | Change proposal is unclear; no evidence of a goal or purpose. No evidence of rationale for the change or rationale presented does not reflect research evidence, changing technologies, local/national guidelines or government targets. |
| Realistic timescale presented which includes a clear statement of what will be different at the end of that timescale with respect to change being undertaken. | 10 | | 0 | Timescale unrealistic or absent. No clear statement of what will be different at the end of the timescale with respect to the change being undertaken. |
| Clear, chronologically sound action plan presented for the change including what needs to be done, by when and who else needs to be involved. Potential problems, resistance or barriers identified with change methods to prevent or overcome these evident. | 25 | | 0 | Action plan not presented or is presented in an illogical order; no evidence of what needs to be done, by when and who else needs to be involved. No problems, resistance or barriers identified and/or no evidence of change methods to overcome these. |
| Evidence of proposals for evaluation of change. | 10 | | 0 | No evidence of proposals for evaluating the change. |
| Logically developed essay, within word limit, correctly referenced using a recognised referencing system. | 10 | | 0 | Essay is illogical, not within word limits, referenced incorrectly and/or recognised referencing system not used. |

# Index